T0176519

New Horizons in Modeling and Simulation
for Social Epidemiology and Public Health

Wiley Series in

Modeling and Simulation

A complete list of the titles in this series appears at the end of this volume.

New Horizons in Modeling and Simulation for Social Epidemiology and Public Health

Daniel Kim

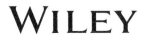

Registered Office
John Wiley & Sons, Inc., 111 River Street, Hoboken, NJ 07030, USA

Editorial Office
111 River Street, Hoboken, NJ 07030, USA

For details of our global editorial offices, customer services, and more information about Wiley products visit us at www.wiley.com.

Wiley also publishes its books in a variety of electronic formats and by print-on-demand. Some content that appears in standard print versions of this book may not be available in other formats.

Library of Congress Cataloging-in-Publication Data

Names: Kim, Daniel (author).
Title: New horizons in modeling and simulation for social epidemiology and public health / Daniel Kim.
Other titles: Wiley series in modeling and simulation.
Description: Hoboken, NJ : Wiley, 2021. | Series: Wiley series in modeling and simulation | Includes bibliographical references and index.
Identifiers: LCCN 2020027470 (print) | LCCN 2020027471 (ebook) | ISBN 9781118589304 (hardback) | ISBN 9781118589427 (Adobe PDF) | ISBN 9781118589571 (epub)
Subjects: MESH: Social Determinants of Health | Public Health | Epidemiologic Methods | Models, Theoretical | Computer Simulation | Social Medicine
Classification: LCC RA418 (print) | LCC RA418 (ebook) | NLM WA 30 | DDC 362.1–dc23
LC record available at https://lccn.loc.gov/2020027470
LC ebook record available at https://lccn.loc.gov/2020027471

Cover Design: Wiley
Cover Images: © vectorfusionart / Shutterstock

Set in 9.5/12.5pt STIXTwoText by SPi Global, Pondicherry, India

SKY10024388_012521

Contents

List of Contributors

Francesco Figari
Department of Economics
University of Insubria
Varese
Italy

Ross A. Hammond
Center on Social Dynamics & Policy
The Brookings Institution
Washington, DC
USA; Brown School
Washington University in St. Louis
St. Louis, MO
USA; and The Santa Fe Institute
Santa Fe, NM
USA

Daniel Kim
Bouvé College of Health Sciences
Northeastern University
Boston, MA
USA; and School of Public Policy and
Urban Affairs
Northeastern University
Boston, MA
USA

Emanuela Lezzi
Department of Economics
University of Insubria
Varese
Italy

Joseph T. Ornstein
Brown School
Washington University in St. Louis
St. Louis, MO
USA

Hilde Philips
Centre for General Practice
University of Antwerp
Antwerpen
Belgium

Gerlinde Verbist
Centre for Social Policy
University of Antwerp
Antwerp
Belgium

Foreword

I am well acquainted with the author of this book *New Horizons in Modeling and Simulation for Social Epidemiology & Public Health*, Dr. Daniel Kim, and the book's contributors including Dr. Ross Hammond. As the former director of the Systems Science Program in the Office of Behavioral and Social Sciences Research (OBSSR) of the National Institutes of Health (NIH), I have had a bird's eye view of this emerging area which I have written extensively about elsewhere (Mabry and Kaplan, 2013; Mabry et al., 2008, 2013).

The NIH and OBSSR have supported a variety of educational opportunities in systems science, such as the Symposia Series on Systems Science and Health (2007; https://www.preventionresearch.org/conferences/training/2007-symposia-series-on-systems-science-and-health/) and the week-long immersion course, *Institute on Systems Science and Health (*ISSH*),* which ran annually from 2009 to 2012. More recently, the NIH has funded short courses such as *Dynamic Systems Science Modeling for Public Health* (PIs: Bruch, Hammond, Osgood; healthmodeling. org). However, one of the noteworthy gaps in the field is adequate instructional material in book form devoted to systems science applications to public health.

In 2012, Drs. Kim and Hammond both participated (Dr. Kim as a trainee and Dr. Hammond as the lead instructor) in the agent-based modeling (ABM) track of the week-long ISSH training course, at Washington University in St. Louis, hosted by Drs. Peter Hovmand and Doug Luke. As a cofounder and producer of ISSH (with Dr. Bobby Milstein, then at Centers for Disease Control and Prevention [CDC]), I had the privilege to witness the germ of this book. Dr. Kim has taken the best he has to offer in the social determinants of health and microsimulation modeling, complemented it with the expertise of Dr. Hammond in ABM and of other excellent book contributors with command of their subject areas, and produced what is destined to become a key resource for public health students, professors, and practitioners. *New Horizons in Modeling and Simulation for Social Epidemiology & Public Health*, with its focus on agent-based modeling, microsimulation, and social determinants of health, is the perfect complement to the recent entrants in this area (El-Sayed and Galea, 2017; Kaplan et al., 2017) as well as Dr. Thomas Valente's (2010) impactful *Social Networks and Health*.

As indicated by its title, *New Horizons in Modeling and Simulation for Social Epidemiology & Public Health* is designed to give graduate students in public health an introduction to modeling and simulation to address research questions in social epidemiology and public health. While this is an excellent resource for this audience, it is sure to become a staple on the bookshelf of not only students but professors in public health and many other health-relevant disciplines. The book provides an excellent introduction to social epidemiology followed by classic case examples in ABM (Schelling model and study of the historic Anasazi population; also within the book's covers the reader will find essential background on ABM use in public health including an overview of ABM for infectious disease modeling, obesity, and tobacco control) and highlights some of the seminal contributions Dr. Hammond has made to the field. The book contains a comprehensive introduction to microsimulation including how to make informed choices regarding time and space, data, policy rules and scope, population structure, validation, and more. An application section illustrates microsimulation models used in population health. A chapter is devoted to educating the reader about various microsimulation models in the social sciences (economics, demography, geography, transportation, and environmental sciences). The book never loses its focus on the social determinants of health, and there are valuable chapters devoted to reviewing the literature on microsimulation models and social determinants of health including important recent contributions by Dr. Kim (Chapter 9), as well as the potential of microsimulation to explore other questions in this vein (Chapter 10). Finally, the book lays out a conceptual model and empirical examples of how ABM and microsimulation can be integrated for additional impact.

With so much information packed into this readable book, it will quickly become a go-to reference and primer of choice for anyone interested in modeling for public health and/or interested in studying the social determinants of health.

Patricia L. Mabry, PhD
Research Investigator
HealthPartners Institute
Former Senior Advisor and Acting Deputy Director, National Institutes of Health (NIH) Office of Behavioral and Social Sciences Research (OBSSR)

References

El-Sayed, A.M. and Galea, S. (eds.) (2017). *Systems Science and Population Health*. Oxford University Press.

Kaplan, G.A., Diez Roux, A.V., and Simon, C.P. (eds.) (2017). *Growing Inequality: Bridging Complex Systems, Population Health, and Health Disparities.* Washington, D.C.: Westphalia Press.

Mabry, P.L. and Kaplan, R.M. (2013). Systems science: a good investment for the public's health. *Health Education and Behavior* 40 (1 suppl): S9–S12.

Mabry, P.L., Milstein, B., Abraido-Lanza, A.F. et al. (2013). Opening a window on systems science research in health promotion and public health. *Health Education and Behavior* 40 (1 suppl): 5S–8S.

Mabry, P.L., Olster, D.H., Morgan, G.D., and Abrams, D.B. (2008). Interdisciplinarity and systems science to improve population health: a view from the NIH office of behavioral and social sciences research. *American Journal of Preventive Medicine* 35 (2 suppl): S211–S224.

Valente, T.W. (2010). *Social Networks and Health: Models, Methods, and Applications*, vol. 1. New York: Oxford University Press.

Acknowledgements

I am grateful to the National Library of Medicine at the United States National Institutes of Health for awarding me a Grant for Scholarly Works in Biomedicine and Health to support the writing of this book (grant number G13 LM012056). I also express my appreciation to Kyle Oddis for editorial assistance. I dedicate this book to my father, Sung Gyum Kim, and to all those in the fields of social epidemiology and public health—past, present and future—who have devoted or will devote their lives to improving population health and health equity for all.

— Daniel Kim, MD, DrPH, Boston, Massachusetts

List of Figures

List of Tables

Part I

Introduction

1

A Primer on the Social Determinants of Health

Daniel Kim

Bouvé College of Health Sciences, Northeastern University, Boston, MA, USA
School of Public Policy and Urban Affairs, Northeastern University, Boston, MA, USA

1.1 Introduction

We begin this book with a simple example of cross-country comparisons of life expectancy that illustrates the striking differences in health across populations. The social determinants of health—fundamental social and economic conditions in which we live, work, and play—may help to shape and explain such stark population health inequalities. In this introductory chapter, I present a conceptual framework for the social determinants of health and two related population health frameworks—the 3 P's (people, places, and policies) Population Health Triad and the Health in All Policies (HiAP) approach. I next discuss approaches for studying the social determinants of health, highlight what we know so far about them, and give some practical examples of their estimated large public health impacts if we were to intervene and modify them.

1.2 The Health Olympics: Winners and Losers

The "Health Olympics" is a term that was coined to describe how rich countries perform relative to each other in life expectancy at birth (Population Health Forum 2003). Figure 1.1 shows these results for 2017 by sex and for the sexes combined based on data for Organisation for Economic Co-operation and Development (OECD) countries (OECD 2018). In these hypothetical Olympics, there are clear winners and losers.

Despite being one of the richest nations in the world, the United States fails to medal in this imaginary international competition; in fact, it falls well short of the podium, placing twenty-seventh, with an overall life expectancy of 78.6 years. By contrast, Japan wins the gold medal for life expectancy for men and women

New Horizons in Modeling and Simulation for Social Epidemiology and Public Health,
First Edition. Daniel Kim.
© 2021 John Wiley & Sons, Inc. Published 2021 by John Wiley & Sons, Inc.

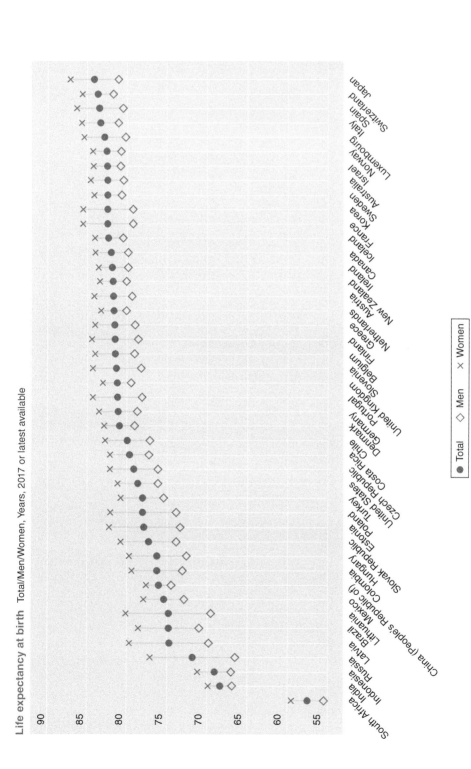

Life expectancy at birth Total/Men/Women, Years, 2017 or latest available

● Total ◇ Men ✕ Women

Figure 1.1   Life expectancy at birth for OECD countries. *Source*: From OECD (2018).

combined at 84.1 years—first among women at 87.1 years, second among men at 81.0 years—and bests the United States by 5.5 years, an enormous gap in life expectancy at a population level. Meanwhile, Australia and a number of countries in the European Union either land on the medal podium or are at least very close to it (Figure 1.1).

Differences in life expectancy at birth are often ascribed to a number of factors, including variations in living standards, lifestyle risk factors, education, and access to health services. But what additional insights can research shed in relation to such patterns? In 2013, the U.S. National Academy of Sciences (NAS) commissioned a scientific panel to explore such cross-national comparisons in life expectancy. This panel released its findings in a report entitled *U.S. Health in International Perspective: Shorter Lives Poorer Health* (National Research Council and Committee on Population 2013). The panel compared health outcomes in the United States to those of 16 comparable high-income countries, including whether the US health disadvantage exists across all ages. It also explored potential explanations and assessed the broader implications of these findings. The panel identified a strikingly consistent and pervasive pattern of higher mortality and worse health among Americans compared to those in other nations between the late 1990s and 2008. This health disadvantage starts at birth, affects all age groups up to age 75, and encompasses multiple health and disease outcomes and conditions (e.g. injuries and homicide, infections, heart disease, obesity, and arthritis) and biological and behavioral risk factors (National Research Council and Committee on Population 2013).

Furthermore, the NAS panel reported that premature deaths occurring before age 50 accounted for as much as two-thirds of the difference in life expectancy in men between the United States and other countries and one-third of the difference in women (National Research Council and Committee on Population 2013). Skyrocketing overdoses of drugs, primarily due to opioids, are a major contributor to these premature deaths (National Center for Health Statistics 2017). These fatal overdoses played a role in declines in life expectancy among Americans for a second consecutive year in 2015 and 2016 (Kochanek et al. 2017), marking the first time this has happened in more than half a century. Gun deaths also rose in 2016 for a second consecutive year. Firearm-related injuries contribute substantially to life expectancy, accounting for 7.1% of premature deaths or years of potential life lost before the age of 65 (Fowler et al. 2015).

Americans reach the age of 50 in worse health than their counterparts in other high-income countries as older adults experience higher levels of morbidity and mortality from chronic diseases. Even socioeconomically advantaged (i.e. college educated or higher income) Americans fare worse than their counterparts in England and other countries (National Research Council and Committee on Population 2013). In offering potential explanations for these patterns, the panel referenced underlying societal factors—which we now commonly refer to as the *social determinants of health*—as possible root causes of the higher levels of morbidity and mortality and shorter life expectancies in the United States (National Research Council and Committee on Population 2013). For instance, despite its vast economy, the United States possesses considerably higher poverty rates and levels of income inequality than most high-income countries. In addition, although the United States once led the world in educational performance, students in many other countries now routinely outperform US students; these findings are analogous to the relative standings of these countries in the Health Olympics. Finally, in contrast to the United States, a number of other countries such as Sweden and Norway in Scandinavia offer larger public welfare and other social safety net programs. Such programs and services could conceivably help residents to better weather the storm of adverse effects on health caused by poor economic and social conditions (Adema et al. 2011; Kim 2016).

1.3 What are the Social Determinants of Health?

In 2005, the World Health Organization (WHO) established a Commission on the Social Determinants of Health that was tasked with the job of supporting countries to address the upstream social factors that shape population health and health inequities (WHO Commission on the Social Determinants of Health 2008). The overall goal of the Commission was to draw the attention of governments and society to the social determinants of health and to create better social conditions for health, particularly amongst the most vulnerable populations. The commission delivered its final report to the WHO in 2008 (WHO Commission on the Social Determinants of Health 2008).

As defined by the WHO Commission, the social determinants of health are "the conditions in which people are born, grow, live, work, and age" (WHO Commission on the Social Determinants of Health 2008). These social determinants extend well beyond the confines of the health care system and include aspects of our neighborhood and workplace environments (e.g. the food, built, and social environments) and the social and economic policies (e.g. tax policies) that govern the regions in which we live. It is these "upstream" nonmedical social determinants that are increasingly understood as the root causes of population health inequalities, even within rich nations (Marmot and Bell 2009; Woolf and Braveman 2011). Such social determinants offer a critical lens to explain why the average life expectancy in America has lagged well behind other nations, despite the fact that the United States remains one of the richest nations in the world and spends more on a per-capita basis on health care than all other developed nations globally (Marmot and Bell 2009). Identifying what impacts various social determinants have on population health is now the central focus of the growing public health field known as social epidemiology.

The WHO Commission on the Social Determinants of Health developed a conceptual framework of the social determinants of health (Solar and Irwin 2007; WHO Commission on the Social Determinants of Health 2008). Figure 1.2 shows an adaptation of this conceptual framework. As illustrated in this figure, the social determinants of health are composed of the material living and working conditions and social environmental conditions in which people are born, live, work, and age, along with the structural drivers of these conditions. These structural drivers include individual- and area-level socioeconomic status (SES), race/ethnicity, residential segregation, gender, social capital/cohesion, and the macroeconomic and macrosocial contexts, e.g. macroeconomic and social policies including labor market regulations (Muntaner et al. 2012), political factors including governance and political rights (Chung and Muntaner 2006; Bezo et al. 2012), and cultural factors. Examples of macroeconomic determinants include the gross domestic product

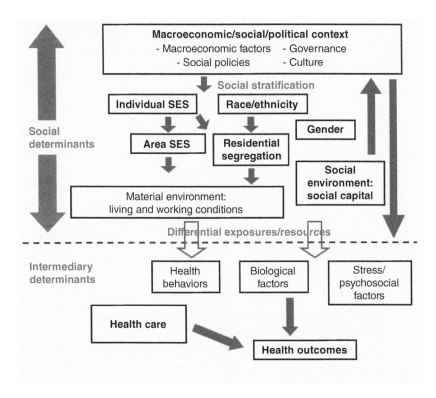

Figure 1.2   A social determinants of health conceptual framework. *Source*: Adapted from Kim and Saada (2013) and Solar and Irwin (2007).

(GDP) per capita and income inequality—the gap between the rich and the poor within societies.

The broader macroeconomic and social context generates social stratification, that is, the sorting of people into dominant and subordinate SES, racial/ethnic, and gender groups (Figure 1.2). Through social stratification and differential exposures of individuals to levels of material factors/social resources, social determinants such as individual/area-level SES, race/ethnicity, and social capital shape individual-level intermediary determinants, including behavioral factors (e.g. maternal smoking), biological factors, and psychosocial factors (e.g. social support), which in turn produce differential risks of, and inequities in, health outcomes (Figure 1.2). Access to health care and the quality of health care are also determinants of these outcomes, yet health care factors are believed to play lesser roles compared to societal factors (Figure 1.2). This is supported by cross-national evidence on health care spending and life expectancy. Moreover, even in societies with a national health system in place (e.g. Canada and the United Kingdom), socioeconomic disparities and gradients in health are salient and well established.

1.4 The 3 P's (people, places, and policies) Population Health Triad

Implicit in this conceptualization of the social determinants of health is that more upstream population characteristics, places, and policies matter to population health. Jointly, we can refer to these three factors that are pivotal to population health as the "3 P's" (people, places, and policies) Population Health Triad (Figure 1.3). The classic Host–Agent–Environment epidemiologic triad posits that a susceptible host, an external agent, and an environment are needed to produce disease. Similarly, both places and policies interact with populations to manifest disease. For example, neighborhoods where we live can influence our health through

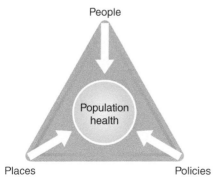

People

Population health

Places   Policies

Figure 1.3   The 3 P's (people, places, and policies) Population Health Triad.

physical and material characteristics such as air quality, access to nutritious foods and opportunities for leisure and exercise, health services, and education/schools and employment opportunities (Braveman et al. 2011). Policies in nonhealth sectors (e.g. transportation, education, and housing) can also intersect with and shape health. Social policies such as those that affect levels of welfare spending and tax policies that determine the rich–poor gap have plausible linkages to the social environment, health behaviors, and individual health and disease endpoints. Reciprocal interactions are also possible, with populations being able to shape both policies and places, such as by mobilizing together through social capital (e.g. political activism) to effect change (Figure 1.2).

To help address the social determinants of health at a government level, in 2010, the WHO and the Government of South Australia (2010) developed the HiAP approach through the Adelaide Statement on HiAP. In this comprehensive population health strategy, health considerations in policymaking permeate and encompass multiple public sectors that may influence health, such as transportation, agriculture, housing and urban development, and education (Figure 1.4). The HiAP approach was founded on the notion that many social determinants of health are outside the purview of public health agencies. The roots of this radical approach can be traced back to the seminal ideas put forth

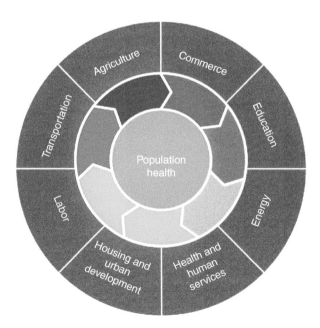

Figure 1.4 Examples of multiple public sectors collectively adopting a Health in All Policies (HiAP) approach.

in the Alma Ata Declaration on Primary Health Care (1978) and the Ottawa Charter for Health Promotion (1986). The HiAP approach became reinforced in the 2011 Rio Political Declaration on Social Determinants of Health (World Health Organization 2016a).

The HiAP approach has been increasingly adopted in jurisdictions around the world. For example, the Department of Housing and Urban Development (HUD) in the United States has embraced a HiAP approach and is collaborating with the U.S. Department of Health and Human Services (HHS) to ensure the integration of the elderly and disabled into the community via housing and human service agencies to enable them to live as long and as healthily as possible (Bostic et al. 2012). HUD further encourages applicants to regional planning and neighborhood initiative grants to incorporate health metrics into their baseline assessments of neighborhoods and asks them to indicate how they will support regional planning efforts that consider public health impacts (Bostic et al. 2012). Moreover, to attain objectives on the social determinants of health, the HiAP approach has been encouraged by Healthy People 2020 (2010), the U.S. Centers for Disease Control and Prevention initiative that establishes national goals and objectives for policy, programs, and activities to address the major health challenges facing our country today. The Secretary's Advisory Committee on Healthy People Objectives for 2020 (Office of Disease Prevention and Health Promotion 2010) has further advised that all federal agencies (e.g. the Departments of Education, Transportation, and HUD) should be required to include Healthy People in their strategic plans.

In 2010, the US state of California created a HiAP Task Force, with representation of 19 state agencies, offices, and departments. Employing a HiAP framework, this statewide effort brought policymakers together to identify and recommend programs, policies, and strategies to improve health, including multiagency initiatives addressing transportation, housing, affordable healthy foods, safe neighborhoods, and green spaces. Additional recommendations included the development of health criteria in the discretionary funding review process and incorporating health issues into statewide data collection and survey efforts (Health in All Policies Task Force 2010).

The region of South Australia has also implemented the HiAP approach. Its HiAP model is based on the twin pillars of central governance and accountability and a "health lens" analysis process, which aims to identify key interactions and synergies between South Australia's Strategic Plan (SASP) targets, policies, and population health (Kickbusch and Buckett 2010). Notably, it was in Adelaide, the capital of South Australia, that the 2010 Adelaide Statement of HiAP was first developed. The South Australian Public Health Act was developed during the early implementation stages of HiAP and provided a legislative mandate to allow HiAP approaches to be systematically adopted across state and local governments within the region (Delany et al. 2015).

To strengthen the overall accountability for the HiAP pledges made by countries in the 2011 Rio Political Declaration on Social Determinants of Health, the WHO is currently developing a global monitoring system for intersectoral interventions on the social determinants of health to improve health equity (World Health Organization 2016b).

1.5 Conventional Approaches to Studying the Social Determinants of Health

Randomized experiments are the gold standard of study designs to establish cause-and-effect relationships. Yet, it is often neither feasible nor ethical to conduct experiments that randomly assign people or places to different levels of social determinants of health. As a result, evidence on the impacts of the social determinants of health has been largely based on observational studies, i.e. ecological, cohort, case–control, and cross-sectional studies. Within such observational studies, traditional epidemiological approaches for studying the impacts of social determinants of health include multivariate analysis, which controls for factors that predict both the social determinants and health outcomes, i.e. so-called potential "confounders."

In addition, studies have explored these relationships by testing for single or multiple factors as potential mediators of the population health impacts of social determinants that could lend plausibility to the presence of causal associations. Because such social determinants are often contextual or area-based factors (e.g. factors at the neighborhood or regional level), multilevel models that incorporate the hierarchical structure of data—such as individuals living within neighborhoods or states—are used to account for similarities and statistical nonindependence of individuals living within the same geographical areas (Goldstein et al. 2002).

1.6 Novel Approaches to Strengthen Causal Inference in Studying the Social Determinants of Health

A growing body of literature is attempting to reduce alternative explanations and other sources of bias in nonexperimental studies on the social determinants of health and more generally within public health. These novel approaches to strengthen causal inference include but are not limited to instrumental variable (IV) analysis, fixed effects analysis, propensity score analysis, inverse probability weighting, and natural experiments. By isolating random variation in the exposure, IV analysis can yield unbiased estimates of the causal association between an exposure and outcome, including through reducing attenuation bias due to measurement error and confounding bias due to both observed and unobserved factors (Kim 2016). Such approaches are increasingly being used to evaluate the causal roles of risk factors in public health, including obesity, neighborhood conditions, the social environment, and state policies (Davey Smith et al. 2009; Fish et al. 2010; Kim et al. 2011; Mojtabai and Crum 2013; Hawkins and Baum 2014; Kim 2016).

Similar to multivariable regression, propensity score analysis can control for imbalances between comparison groups and can thereby control for confounding. It has the advantage of being more efficient than traditional regression when there are relatively fewer events (Cepeda et al. 2003). However, like multivariable regression, propensity score analysis cannot control for unobserved or unmeasured confounders. Inverse probability weighting has also been used as an approach to estimate the counterfactual or potential outcome if all subjects were assigned to either exposure/treatment (Mansournia and Altman 2016). Finally, natural experiments or other quasi-experimental designs such as regression discontinuity designs (Moscoe et al. 2015) can exploit random variation in exposures as in an experimental study and can thereby minimize confounding due to both observed and unobserved factors as a source of bias.

Results from individual studies can also be qualitatively reviewed in aggregate to identify existing gaps in methodological approaches, potential sources of bias, and similarities/differences in their results. Results across studies can be quantitatively summarized in meta-analyses that yield overall point estimates of exposure–outcome associations, although, importantly, such estimates are only as good as the quality of the studies that are included in the meta-analyses (Egger et al. 2001).

1.7 What Do We Know About the Social Determinants of Health?

As Bambra et al. (2010) have noted, there are clear limitations to the existing evidence based on the social determinants of health. First, observational studies that dominate the literature can only hint at possible interventions and their associated health effects; causal inference is an inherent limitation. Second, there is still only sparse evidence on the impacts of interventions on the social determinants of health. Bambra et al. (2010) conducted an "umbrella review" of the existing systematic reviews of the evidence on specific interventions on the social determinants of health spanning housing/living environment, work environment, transportation, health and social care services, agriculture and food, and water and sanitation. They identified some suggestive evidence that certain categories of interventions may impact inequalities regarding the health of specific disadvantaged groups, particularly in the fields of housing and work environment. Yet in other areas, such as evidence on policies in education, the health system, food and agriculture, and more generally on the influences of macro-level policies on health inequalities, the empirical literature on interventions was more limited (Bambra et al. 2010).

In a more recent umbrella review, Thomson et al. (2017) adopted a systematic review approach to summarize the state of knowledge on how public health policy interventions (e.g. taxation and educational campaigns) may impact health inequalities such as differential effects across socioeconomic groups or effects of interventions targeted at disadvantaged groups. After searching studies published up to May 2017 within 20 databases (e.g. Medline, EMBASE, CINAHL, PsycINFO, Social Science Citation Index, Sociological Abstracts, and the Cochrane Library), the authors identified 24 systematic reviews reporting 128 relevant primary studies. They then summarized the evidence on policies (fiscal, regulation, education, preventive treatment, and screening) across eight public health domains (tobacco; food and nutrition; the control of infectious diseases; screening; road traffic injuries; air, land, and water pollution; built environment; and workplace regulations). The systematic reviews were mixed in quality, and the results were mixed across public health domains. For the tobacco, food and nutrition, and control of infectious diseases domains, the authors found evidence to suggest that fiscal and regulation policies were more beneficial for reducing or preventing health inequalities than educational campaigns (Thomson et al. 2017).

1.8 How Addressing the Social Determinants of Health Could Change Lives

In principle, intervening on the social determinants of health should have profound effects on population health outcomes and health equity. These outcomes include the numbers of lives saved and the occurrence of disease and other morbidity outcomes such as Disability-Adjusted Life Years (DALYs) (Murray et al. 2015). If we consider the distal nature of these social determinants in Figure 1.2, the impacts of these determinants on population health may in fact be stronger than those of proximal biological and behavioral factors at the individual level (such as smoking and high cholesterol), because upstream social determinants likely shape many of these biological and behavioral factors.

Yet what does the empirical evidence show about the impacts of social determinants of health at a population level? Drawing on studies from the public health literature, the numbers of adult deaths attributable to six social determinants of health have been estimated (Galea et al., 2011): low education, poverty, low social support, area-level poverty, income inequality, and racial segregation. The investigators calculated summary relative risk estimates of mortality, and used prevalence estimates for each of these social determinants to estimate the associated population attributable risks (PARs, the percentage of deaths attributed to each factor), and then project the total number of deaths attributable to each social determinant in the United States. Through this approach, the authors estimated that 245 000 deaths would have taken place among Americans in the year 2000 due to low education, 176 000 deaths to racial segregation, 162 000 deaths to low social support, 133 000 deaths to individual poverty, 119 000 deaths to income inequality, and 39 000 deaths to area-level poverty. These estimates due to social determinants of health were comparable to the total numbers of deaths due to the leading pathophysiological causes such as heart attacks (192 898 deaths), strokes (167 661 deaths), and lung cancer (155 521 deaths) (Galea et al. 2011). To further put the size of these numbers into perspective, in the year 2000, it was estimated that smoking resulted in 269 655 deaths among men and 173 940 deaths among women in the United States (Centers for Disease Control and Prevention (CDC) 2008).

In another study, Krueger et al. (2015) estimated the mortality attributable to education under three hypothetical scenarios: (i) individuals having less than a high school degree, (ii) individuals having some college education but not completing a bachelor's degree, and (iii) individuals having any level of education but not completing a bachelor's degree. The authors used National Health Interview Survey data (1986–2004) linked to prospective mortality through 2006 and discrete-time survival models to derive annual attributable mortality estimates. The estimated numbers of attributable deaths were striking: 45 243 deaths in the 2010 US population were attributed to individuals having less than a high school degree rather than a high school degree; 110 068 deaths were due to individuals having some college education; and 554 525 deaths were attributed to individuals having anything less than a bachelor's degree but not a bachelor's degree (Krueger et al. 2015). The total numbers of deaths due to having less than a high school degree was similar among women and men and among non-Hispanic Blacks and Whites and was greater for cardiovascular disease than for cancer. Overall, these estimates point to the substantial impacts that policies that increase educational opportunities could have on reducing the burden of adult mortality (Krueger et al. 2015).

Using nationally-representative data, Kim (2016) estimated the impacts of state and local spending on welfare and education on the risks of dying from major causes. Each additional $250 per capita spent on welfare predicted a 3-percentage point lower probability of dying from any cause, and each additional $250 per capita spent on welfare and education predicted a 1.6-percentage point lower probability and a nearly 1-percentage point lower probability of dying from coronary heart disease (CHD). To put such numbers into context, these changes are on the order of reductions achieved through treating a patient with high blood pressure or cholesterol—representing clinically meaningful changes (Kim 2016).

In a cross-national study that implemented IV analysis to enhance causal inference, Kim et al. (2011) further estimated the population health impacts of raising social capital across 40 countries. Among those aged 15–74 years in 40 nations with at least 40% of the country trusting of others, raising country percentages of social trust by 20 percentage points in countries with at least 30% of a country's citizens trusting of others and by 10 percentage points in countries with 30–40% average country trust was predicted to avert nearly 287 000 deaths per year.

Finally, Kondo et al. (2009) conducted a meta-analysis of cohort studies including roughly 60 million participants in which people living in regions with high-income inequality had an excess risk for premature mortality independent of their SES, age, and sex. The estimated excess mortality risk was 8% for each 0.05 unit increase in the Gini coefficient (a common measure of income inequality theoretically ranging from 0, representing perfect equality, to 1, corresponding to perfect inequality). While this excess risk appears modest, all of society is exposed to income inequality, such that the aggregate effects can be significant (Kondo et al. 2009). The authors estimated that if the inequality–mortality relation is truly causal, more than 1.5 million deaths (9.6% of total adult mortality in the 15–60 age group) could be averted in 30 OECD countries by reducing the Gini coefficient to below the threshold value of 0.3 (Kondo et al. 2009).

Notably, according to Figure 1.2, there should also be substantial impacts of intervening on the social determinants of health on health inequities across population groups, as defined along social axes such as gender, race/ethnicity, and SES. For example, government spending on public assistance programs (e.g. Aid to Families with Dependent Children) and tax credit programs (e.g. the Earned Income Tax Credit) should reduce income disparities between the rich and the poor and thereby reduce associated gaps in health, since income is a strong determinant of health and disease.

As the U.S. National Academy of Sciences panel concluded in its report, if the United States fails to address its growing health disadvantage in the near future, it will lag even further behind comparable countries in life expectancy and across a wide range of other population health outcomes. By adversely affecting the productivity of the workforce through worse population health, the economy of the United States would also continue to suffer, whereas other countries would continue to reap the economic benefits of having healthier populations. Because of how much is at stake, the panel concluded that it would hence be at the United States' peril that it continue to ignore its growing health disadvantage (National Research Council and Committee on Population 2013). Meanwhile, other countries will still need to maintain their efforts on addressing the social determinants of health if they wish to sustain and/or improve their relative standings in the Health Olympics.

Overall, the findings summarized in this chapter make a strong case for intervening at the policy level on social determinants to improve population health and reduce population health inequities. It is also clear that much more empirical evidence is needed if we wish to establish the population health impacts of the social determinants of health. These evidence gaps include estimates of the effects of social determinants of health on the incidence of diseases and on morbidity outcomes such as DALYs; the estimated population-wide health impacts of intervening on the social determinants of health through scaled-up interventions and policies; and economic evaluations (e.g. cost-effectiveness) of such interventions.

In the next chapter, we move beyond traditional analytic approaches to provide a rationale for the use of systems science methods. In particular, we introduce two major sets of analytical tools for modeling and simulating impacts of the social determinants of health: agent-based modeling and microsimulation models. These two novel system science tools and their growing applications in social epidemiology and public health form the primary substance of this book.

References

Adema, W., Fron, P., and Ladaique, M. (2011). Is the European welfare state really more expensive?: indicators on social spending, 1980–2012; and a manual to the OECD social expenditure database (SOCX). OECD Social, Employment and Migration working papers, No. 124, OECD Publishing.

Bambra, C., Gibson, M., Amanda, S. et al. (2010). Tackling the wider social determinants of health and health inequalities: evidence from systematic reviews. *Journal of Epidemiology and Community Health* 64: 284–291.

Bezo, B., Maggi, S., and Roberts, W.L. (2012). The rights and freedoms gradient of health: evidence from a cross-national study. *Frontiers in Psychology* 3: 441.

Bostic, R.W., Thornton, R.L.J., Rudd, E.C., and Sternthal, M.J. (2012). Health in all policies: the role of the US Department of Housing and Urban Development and present and future challenges. *Health Affairs* 31: 2130–2137.

Braveman, P., Egerter, S., and Williams, D.R. (2011). The social determinants of health: coming of age. *Annual Review of Public Health* 32: 381–398.

Centers for Disease Control and Prevention (CDC) (2008). Smoking-attributable mortality, years of potential life lost, and productivity losses-United States, 2000–2004. *Morbidity and Mortality Weekly Report* 57: 1226–1228.

Cepeda, M.S., Boston, R., Farrar, J.T., and Strom, B.L. (2003). Comparison of logistic regression versus propensity score when the number of events is low and there are multiple confounders. *American Journal of Epidemiology* 158 (3): 280–287.

Charter, O. (1986, November). Ottawa Charter for health promotion. In *First International Conference on Health Promotion*, pp. 17–21.

Chung, H. and Muntaner, C. (2006). Political and welfare state determinants of infant and child health indicators: an analysis of wealthy countries. *Social Science and Medicine* 63: 829–842.

Davey Smith, G., Sterne, J.A.C., Fraser, A. et al. (2009). The associatiodczcn between BMI and mortality using offspring BMI as an indicator of own BMI: large intergenerational mortality study. *British Medical Journal* 339: b5043.

Declaration of Alma-Ata. (1978). Pan American Health Organization. https://www.paho.org/English/DD/PIN/alma-ata_declaration.htm (accessed 1 July 2019).

Delany, T., Lawless, A., Baum, F. et al. (2015). Health in all policies in South Australia: what has supported early implementation? *Health Promotion International* 31 (4): 888–898.

Egger, M., Smith, G.D., and Sterne, J.A. (2001). Uses and abuses of meta-analysis. *Clinical Medicine* 1 (6): 478–484.

Fish, J.S., Ettner, S., Ang, A. et al. (2010). Association of perceived neighborhood safety on body mass index. *American Journal of Public Health* 100: 2296–2303.

Fowler, K.A., Dahlberg, L.L., Haileyesus, T., and Annest, J.L. (2015). Firearm injuries in the United States. *Preventive Medicine* 79: 5–14.

Galea, S., Tracy, M., Hoggatt, K.J. et al. (2011). Estimated deaths attributable to social factors in the United States. *American Journal of Public Health* 101: 1456–1465.

Goldstein, H., Browne, W., and Rasbash, J. (2002). Multilevel modeling of medical data. *Statistics in Medicine* 21 (21): 3291–3315.

Hawkins, S.S. and Baum, C. (2014). Impact of state cigarette taxes on disparities in maternal smoking during pregnancy. *American Journal of Public Health* 104 (8): 1464–1470.

Health in All Policies Task Force (2010). *Health in All Policies Task Force Report to the Strategic Growth Council Executive Summary*. Sacramento: Health in All Policies Task Force.

Kickbusch, I. and Buckett, K. (eds.) (2010). *Implementing Health in All Policies: Adelaide 2010*. Adelaide: Health in All Policies Unit, Department of Health; Government of South Australia.

Kim, D. (2016). The associations between US state and local social spending, income inequality, and individual all-cause and cause-specific mortality: the National Longitudinal Mortality Study. *Preventive Medicine* 84: 62–68.

Kim, D. and Saada, A. (2013). The social determinants of infant mortality and birth outcomes in western developed nations: a cross-country systematic review. *International Journal of Environmental Research and Public Health* 10: 2296–2335.

Kim, D., Baum, C.F., Ganz, M.L. et al. (2011). The contextual effects of social capital on health: a cross-national instrumental variable analysis. *Social Science and Medicine* 73: 1689–1697.

Kochanek, K.D., Murphy, S.L., Xu, J.Q., and Arias, E. (2017). *Mortality in the United States, 2016. NCHS Data Brief, no 293*. Hyattsville, MD: National Center for Health Statistics.

Kondo, N., Sembajwe, G., Kawachi, I. et al. (2009). Income inequality, mortality, and self rated health: meta-analysis of multilevel studies. *British Medical Journal* 339: b4471.

Krueger, P.M., Tran, M.K., Hummer, R.A., and Chang, V.W. (2015). Mortality attributable to low levels of education in the United States. *PlOS ONE* 10 (7): e0131809.

Mansournia, M.A. and Altman, D.G. (2016). Inverse probability weighting. *BMJ* 352: 189.

Marmot, M.G. and Bell, R. (2009). Action on health disparities in the United States: commission on Social Determinants of Health. *Journal of the American Medical Association* 301 (11): 1169–1171.

Mojtabai, R. and Crum, R.M. (2013). Cigarette smoking and onset of mood and anxiety disorders. *American Journal of Public Health* 103: 1656–1665.

Moscoe, E., Bor, J., and Bärnighausen, T. (2015). Regression discontinuity designs are underutilized in medicine, epidemiology, and public health: a review of current and best practice. *Journal of Clinical Epidemiology* 68 (2): 122–133.

Muntaner, C., Chung, H., Benach, J., and Ng, E. (2012). Hierarchical cluster analysis of labour market regulations and population health: a taxonomy of low- and middle-income countries. *BMC Public Health* 12: 286.

Murray, C.J., Barber, R.M., Foreman, K.J. et al. (2015). Global, regional, and national disability-adjusted life years (DALYs) for 306 acute diseases and injuries and healthy life expectancy (HALE) for 188 countries, 1990–2013: quantifying the epidemiological transition. *The Lancet* 386 (10009): 2145–2191.

National Center for Health Statistics (2017). Provisional counts of drug overdose deaths. https://www.cdc.gov/nchs/data/health_policy/monthly-drug-overdose-death-estimates.pdf (accessed 6 August 2017).

National Research Council and Committee on Population (2013). *US Health in International Perspective: Shorter Lives, Poorer Health*. Washington, DC: National Academies Press.

OECD (2018). Life expectancy at birth (indicator). DOI: https://doi.org/10.1787/27e0fc9d-en

Office of Disease Prevention and Health Promotion (2010). *Healthy People 2020*. Washington, DC: U.S. Department of Health and Human Services, Office of Disease Prevention and Health Promotion.

Population Health Forum (2003). http://depts.washington.edu/eqhlth/ (accessed 1 July 2019).

Solar, O. and Irwin, A. (2007). A conceptual framework for action on the social determinants of health. Discussion Paper for the Commission on Social Determinants of Health. World Health Organization, Geneva.

Thomson, K., Hillier-Brown, F., Todd, A. et al. (2017). The effects of public health policies on health inequalities: a review of reviews. *The Lancet* 390: S12.

WHO and the Government of South Australia (2010). The Adelaide Statement on Health in All Policies: moving towards a shared governance for health and well-being. *Health Promotion International* 25 (2): 258–260.

WHO Commission on the Social Determinants of Health (2008). *Closing the Gap in a Generation: Health Equity through Action on the Social Determinants of Health. Final Report of the Commission on Social Determinants of Health.* Geneva: World Health Organization.

Woolf, S.H. and Braveman, P. (2011). Where health disparities begin: the role of social and economic determinants – and why current policies may make matters worse. *Health Affairs* 30 (10): 1852–1859.

World Health Organization (2016a). *Rio Political Declaration on Social Determinants of Health, 2011.* Brazil: World Health Organization.

World Health Organization (2016b). *Global Monitoring of Action on the Social Determinants of Health: a Proposed Framework and Basket of Core Indicators.* Geneva: World Health Organization.

2

Rationale for New Modeling and Simulation Tools

Agent-Based Modeling and Microsimulation

Daniel Kim[1,2] and Ross A. Hammond[3,4,5]

[1] *Bouvé College of Health Sciences, Northeastern University, Boston, MA, USA*
[2] *School of Public Policy and Urban Affairs, Northeastern University, Boston, MA, USA*
[3] *Center on Social Dynamics & Policy, The Brookings Institution, Washington, DC, USA*
[4] *Brown School, Washington University in St. Louis, St. Louis, MO, USA*
[5] *The Santa Fe Institute, Santa Fe, NM, USA*

2.1 Advantages of Systems Science Approaches over Conventional Approaches

The real world is made up of a series of complex systems. As we have seen in Chapter 1, health and disease are products of causal factors operating through multiple pathways at multiple levels. Such complex systems are not simply linear—they are characterized by causal feedback loops and complex interactions between actors at multiple levels and are inherently dynamic. Traditional multivariable models adopt a more reductionist approach and lack the ability to capture such features. In general, they implement static or discretely longitudinal analyses, do not incorporate potential nonlinearities such as feedback loops, and do not capture behavioral responses of individuals (Luke and Stamatakis 2012). By contrast, systems science approaches were explicitly developed to account for such features.

Although variation in the relationship between exposures and outcomes that is "exogenous" or "as if random" is the primary objective of advanced methods used to strengthen causal inference, the real world is filled with endogeneity. Endogenous factors are those found within the same system, meaning that they may bias the association between an exposure and an outcome. Notably, systems science approaches do not regard the endogeneity of the real world as nuisances; rather, through a more holistic approach, they model the presence of such complex pathways and mechanisms to better understand them (Luke and Stamatakis 2012).

Systems science approaches represent innovative sets of tools that can model and simulate the real world with enough complexity to be useful. Yet importantly, like their traditional model cousins, they reflect simplified versions of reality.

Ideally, systems models retain enough of the salient characteristics of complexity to enhance our understanding of the problem under study, without being so complex themselves that they are opaque and as impenetrable to our understanding as reality itself. Moreover, systems science approaches enable virtual conduct of experiments that are often not feasible, whether due to cost, ethical reasons, or the simple fact that there is no way to explore the impact of an intervention (e.g. policy) and also go back in time and intervene differently to compare outcomes. With simulation models, it is straightforward to compare a wide array of hypothetical scenarios in silico. For further exposition of the virtues of modeling, see Epstein (2008) and Mabry et al. (2010).

2.2   Specific Advantages of Agent-Based Modeling and Microsimulation Modeling

Agent-Based Modeling

Agent-based modeling (ABM) offers four specific advantages for public health research. First, because each actor in the system under study can be explicitly represented, no aggregation or statistical summary is required in treatment of either individual characteristics or outcomes. As a result, ABM is a powerful tool for considering heterogeneity—whether in biology, cognition, demography, or context. This is especially important for topics such as health disparities (Kaplan et al. 2017). Second, ABM offers an effective way to consider adaptation—processes of learning, evolution, or bidirectional interaction between individuals over time. This means that not only can we consider short-run impacts of policies or interventions, but we can also explore potential impacts over very long time horizons. Topics such as obesity, antibiotic resistance, and developmental origins of health and disease often benefit from such considerations. Third, ABM is able to incorporate very sophisticated representations of structure and space, including social network data, physical space data from geographic information systems (GISs) or light detection and ranging (LIDAR), and biological space (e.g. physiology). Rather than either assuming away spatial elements or reducing them to summary statistics (for example, zip code-level density of retailers), agent-based models can carry a full accounting of spatial exposure and interaction throughout the dynamic simulation. Recent efforts to consider "precision prevention" in communities (Gillman and Hammond 2016; Economos and Hammond 2017) and retailer-oriented tobacco control policies (Luke et al. 2017) leverage this facility of ABM. Finally, ABM is well suited for multilevel modeling. Each individual agent can contain detailed representations of "below-the-skin" processes such as energy balance, cognition, decision-making, or disease progression; at the same time, the agents can interact with each other, with physical environments, and with population-level signals (Hammond 2009; Hammond and Ornstein 2014). Although arguably essential to full understanding of many chronic disease challenges, crossing the "skin barrier" remains rare in social epidemiology.

Microsimulation Models

Microsimulation models (MSM) enable simulations of policies on samples of economic agents (individual, households, and firms) at the individual level (Bourguignon and Spadaro 2006). These simulations allow for the projection of the consequences of modifying economic conditions for each individual agent in the sample. Through such projections, we can estimate the overall aggregate impacts of a policy as well as the distributional consequences of the policy in terms of "winners" and "losers." These could be population subgroups as defined by social axes including age, gender, race/ethnicity, and socioeconomic status. Such policies may be expensive and not readily feasible to undertake in the real world. For example, changing the income tax structure can alter what absolute income individuals in a population receive and influence the distribution of income (i.e. levels of income inequality) within the population. Through tax microsimulation, we can hence project the absolute and relative income impacts without actually implementing these changes in the real world. MSM can thus offer a convenient and inexpensive means to estimate the overall population impacts of social policies.

Other Complex Systems Modeling Tools

Other key systems science approaches (not reviewed in this book) include system dynamics models and social network analysis (SNA). System dynamics models differ from ABM and MSM by aggregating factors and their interactions within endogenous systems to better understand high-level phenomena such as the impacts of interventions and policies and their unintended consequences (Homer and Hirsch 2006). SNA studies the relationships between actors and entities—be they individuals, organizations, or countries. Like ABM, SNA can be useful in telescoping between the micro (individual) and the macroscales of analysis; yet unlike ABM, SNA does not always include dynamic simulation nor account for adaptation. Some forms of SNA overlap with ABM. SNA is widely used for understanding the transmission of infectious diseases such as HIV/AIDS and influenza, and the contagion of behaviors such as obesity and depression, since each of these can be transmitted socially (Christakis and Fowler 2007).

2.3 Comparison of Agent-Based and Microsimulation Models

Figure 2.1 illustrates some key differences between ABM, MSM, and statistical models (e.g. regression) as commonly used in population health. Unlike traditional models which draw on existing observational data, system science approaches such as ABM and MSM conduct ex ante assessments—for example, to consider the potential effects of policy interventions for which no data yet exist (and which therefore cannot easily be addressed by linear regression). In doing so, they leverage an ability to account for dynamic histories of individual agents, thereby incorporating changes in exposures over time, and to account for heterogeneous actors and behavioral responses. Behavioral responses include changes in the behaviors of agents in response to a new economic policy (e.g. tax policy) that imposes changes in individuals' budget constraints. Microsimulation is particularly well suited for studying the impacts of economic policies, including tax and welfare policies. Meanwhile, neither ABM nor MSM are specifically designed to enhance causal inference—such as by removing endogeneity—unlike advanced epidemiologic methods such as marginal structural regression and inverse probability weighting approaches that have been developed in recent years (Hernan and Robins 2010).

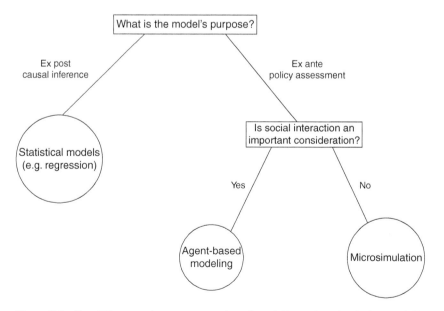

Figure 2.1 Key differences between agent-based modeling, microsimulation modeling, and traditional statistical models.

An important distinction between ABM and MSM as commonly used in population health and social science is that MSM generally do not include any characterization of social interactions between individuals (except indirectly via a social-level variable). By contrast, ABM models are generally focused on such interactions. Hence, MSM might be best suited for, say, consideration of tax policy, whereas ABM might be better suited for studying contagion of infectious disease.

2.4 Why ABM and MSM are Useful for Studying the Social Determinants of Health

In both of the fields of social epidemiology and social policy, understanding the nature of these relationships (such as the effect of a particular social determinant on health) using traditional models is greatly limited by the lack of consideration of the complexity of systems. In order to delineate the true effects of the social determinants of health within the complex systems of entire societies—characterized by multiple agents, nonlinearities, and complex feedback loops—novel modeling and simulation tools such as ABM and MSM are often required. For example, simulation studies can model the intergenerational transmission of socioeconomic disadvantage, an inquiry that is impractical in more traditional studies. Importantly, systems science approaches such as ABM and MSM can enable exploration of the possible impacts of policy options before actually implementing them (Maglio and Mabry 2011), which can avoid the ethical and feasibility issues that can arise from implementing interventions in real life. For example, in the review of the evidence-based interventions for the social determinants of health by Bambra et al. (2010) described in the last chapter, no intervention studies on income inequality were found. Through MSM, we can readily simulate the potential health effects of a tax policy that modifies the income distribution within a population.

The systems science approaches emerging in social epidemiology and public health research today are hardly new. Their historical use dates back to several decades within other disciplines, including physics, economics, engineering, and systems biology (Mabry et al. 2010). For example, systems science approaches such as ABM and MSM have been previously used to address wide-ranging topics such as overfishing, the decline of ancient civilizations, climate change, and terrorism networks (Mabry et al. 2010). Their recent adoption into the public health arena can be attributed to a growing recognition of their utility for addressing intractable public health problems such as the spreading obesity epidemic (Hammond 2009) and the complexity of tobacco control policies (Tengs et al. 2001; Levy et al. 2002). Other recent applications of ABM to population health include analyzing the spread of infectious disease epidemics such as pandemic flu

(Longini et al. 2005); modeling the social determinants of behaviors such as alcohol and drug use (Hoffer et al. 2009); and simulating dynamics of chronic diseases such as diabetes at a population level (Jones et al. 2006).

As should become evident throughout the remainder of this book, the possible applications of ABM and MSM to the social and economic determinants of population health are vast. These potential applications range from studying the spread of infectious diseases (e.g. COVID-19) or spread of intractable problems such as the obesity epidemic, to modeling the social determinants of behaviors such as alcohol or drug use, to simulating the public health impacts of enacting new tax policies. These techniques have been largely developed and applied in other fields including computer science, political science, economics, and social policy. Diffusion and adoption of these approaches into the fields of social epidemiology and public health are more recent, and there remains a tremendous potential for transforming the landscape of these fields by integrating these novel applications.

2.5   Structure of this Book

In this introductory section (Part I), Chapter 1 defines the social determinants of health, discusses conventional approaches for studying them, and indicates the methodological limitations in identifying their impacts and comments on the public health significance of addressing the social determinants of health. In Chapter 2, we have provided a rationale and overview of current concepts and methods for applying two major sets of analytical tools, ABM and MSM, considered within a larger toolkit of modeling and simulation approaches, to study these social determinants.

In the next section, Part II (Chapters 3–6), we focus on conceptual and empirical applications of ABM to help "unpack" our understanding of the social determinants of health. It consists of four chapters providing an overview of current concepts and methods used for ABM and provides a state-of-the-art, critical synthesis of the ABM evidence base both in the social sciences and in social epidemiology on the social determinants of health to inform future public health research and practice.

Chapter 3 reviews the key terms for agent-based models in practitioner language, highlights ABM methods to assess the social determinants of health at a population level, discusses applications for studying the social determinants of health and novel extensions of this methodology, and provides an illustrative example. Chapter 4 gives detailed examples of empirically powerful applications of ABM in the social sciences, including a foundation to inform the more recent ABM evidence on the social determinants of health that are reviewed in the subsequent chapter. This body of evidence is explored and grouped into three key areas: neighborhood research (e.g. residential preferences), research on scaling laws in social systems, and anthropological models. Chapter 5 reviews the current evidence on the applications of ABM in social epidemiology and public health to better understand the impacts of the social determinants of health. This evidence is explored and grouped into three key areas: health disparities, obesity, and tobacco control. Several examples of public health applications of ABM including for modeling obesity and tobacco use are introduced. These include models that explore the effects of social influence on obesity dynamics (Hammond and Ornstein 2014), models of residential segregation and obesity disparities (Auchincloss et al. 2011), and a model examining retail point-of-sale interventions for tobacco control (Luke et al. 2017).

Chapter 6 summarizes the evidence highlighted in Chapters 4 and 5 and past public policy translation of this evidence and discusses the apparent evidence gaps that, if addressed, would advance the ABM field of inquiry for modeling and "unpacking" the social determinants of health.

Part III (Chapters 7–10) analogously focuses on conceptual and empirical applications of MSM to simulate and thus enhance our understanding of the impacts of the social determinants of health. It provides an overview of the current concepts and methods used for MSM and gives a rich synthesis of the MSM evidence base both in the social sciences and in the field of public health on the social determinants of health.

Chapter 7 reviews the key terms using MSM in practitioner language, highlights microsimulation modeling methods to assess the social determinants of health at a population level, discusses applications for studying the social determinants of health and novel extensions of this methodology, and provides an illustrative example. Chapter 8 reviews the current evidence on the applications of MSM in the social sciences and gives a foundation to inform the more recent MSM evidence on the social determinants of health reviewed in the subsequent chapter. Chapter 9 systematically reviews the current evidence on the applications of MSM to better understand the impacts of the social determinants of health. For example, the chapter describes published examples of applications of MSM including projections of the economic cost savings and population health benefits that would occur if the WHO's recommendations on the social determinants of health were to be adopted in Australia and the impacts on mortality burden of modifying US federal income tax policies based on recent proposals. This chapter also highlights some MSM applications to the study of health care policies, disease microsimulation, and health behavior-related policies.

Chapter 10 summarizes the evidence presented in Chapters 8 and 9, comments on public policy translation of some of this evidence, and discusses current evidence gaps that, if filled, could move the MSM field toward a richer understanding of the social determinants of health.

We conclude the book with Part IV, Chapter 11, by discussing the future directions for research using ABM and microsimulation modeling and simulation, including the convergence of aspects of both ABM and MSM into the same analyses. It also comments on facilitators and constraints for the continued emergence of these forms of modeling and simulation and casts light on the potential policy implications of findings from these more complex and integrative models.

References

Auchincloss, A.H., Riolo, R.L., Brown, D.G. et al. (2011). An agent-based model of income inequalities in diet in the context of residential segregation. *American Journal of Preventive Medicine* 40 (3): 303–311.

Bambra, C., Gibson, M., Amanda, S. et al. (2010). Tackling the wider social determinants of health and health inequalities: evidence from systematic reviews. *Journal of Epidemiology and Community Health* 64: 284–291.

Bourguignon, F. and Spadaro, A. (2006). Microsimulation as a tool for evaluating redistribution policies. *The Journal of Economic Inequality* 4 (1): 77–106.

Christakis, N.A. and Fowler, J.H. (2007). The spread of obesity in a large social network over 32 years. *New England Journal of Medicine* 357 (4): 370–379.

Economos, C.D. and Hammond, R.A. (2017). Designing effective and sustainable multifaceted interventions for obesity prevention and healthy communities. *Obesity* 25 (7): 1155–1156.

Epstein, J.M. (2008). Why model? *Journal of Artificial Societies and Social Simulation* 11 (4): 12.

Gillman, M.W. and Hammond, R.A. (2016). Precision treatment and precision prevention: integrating "below and above the skin". *JAMA Pediatrics* 170 (1): 9–10.

Hammond, R.A. (2009). Complex systems modeling for obesity research. *Preventing Chronic Disease* 6 (3): A97.

Hammond, R.A. and Ornstein, J. (2014). A model of social influence on body weight. *Annals of the New York Academy of Sciences* 1331: 34–42.

Hernan, M.A. and Robins, J.M. (2010). *Causal Inference*. Boca Raton, FL: CRC.

Hoffer, L.D., Bobashev, G., and Morris, R.J. (2009). Researching a local heroin market as a complex adaptive system. *American Journal of Community Psychology* 44 (3–4): 273–286.

Homer, J.B. and Hirsch, G.B. (2006). System dynamics modeling for public health: background and opportunities. *American Journal of Public Health* 96 (3): 452–458.

Jones, A.P., Homer, J.B., Murphy, D.L. et al. (2006). Understanding diabetes population dynamics through simulation modeling and experimentation. *American Journal of Public Health* 96 (3): 488–494.

Kaplan, G.A., Roux, A.V.D., Simon, C.P., and Galea, S. (eds.) (2017). *Growing Inequality*. Westphalia Press.

Levy, D.T., Chaloupka, F., Gitchell, J. et al. (2002). The use of simulation models for the surveillance, justification and understanding of tobacco control policies. *Health Care Management Science* 5 (2): 113–120.

Longini, I.M., Nizam, A., Xu, S. et al. (2005). Containing pandemic influenza at the source. *Science* 309 (5737): 1083–1087.

Luke, D.A. and Stamatakis, K.A. (2012). Systems science methods in public health: dynamics, networks, and agents. *Annual Review of Public Health* 33: 357–376.

Luke, D.A., Hammond, R.A., Combs, T. et al. (2017). Tobacco town: computational modeling of policy options to reduce tobacco retailer density. *American Journal of Public Health* 107 (5): 740–746.

Mabry, P.L., Marcus, S.E., Clark, P.I. et al. (2010). Systems science: a revolution in public health policy research. *American Journal of Public Health* 100 (7): 1161–1163.

Maglio, P.P. and Mabry, P.L. (2011). Agent-based models and systems science approaches to public health. *American Journal of Preventive Medicine* 40 (3): 392–394.

Tengs, T.O., Osgood, N.D., and Lin, T.H. (2001). Public health impact of changes in smoking behavior: results from the tobacco policy model. *Medical Care* 39 (10): 1131–1141.

Part II

Agent-Based Modeling

3

Overview of Current Concepts and Process for Agent-Based Modeling

Ross A. Hammond

Center on Social Dynamics & Policy, The Brookings Institution, Washington, DC, USA
Brown School, Washington University in St. Louis, St. Louis, MO, USA
The Santa Fe Institute, Santa Fe, NM, USA

This chapter builds on the brief introduction to agent-based modeling (ABM) provided earlier in the book, explicating in more detail the key terms used to describe ABMs, the key steps in the process of developing and using ABMs as part of a scientific enterprise, and a brief history of the use of agent-based models across scientific fields to date. Later in this section of the book, more detailed expositions of the use of ABMs to solve empirical puzzles in the fields which triangulate social determinants of health (social science and public health) will be provided, along with some discussion of the use of ABMs to inform policy. The chapter is intended to give an overview of the key elements and best practices involved in this type of work; it is not intended as a "how-to" textbook, as training in ABM takes extensive study beyond what is covered here.

3.1 The Components of an Agent-Based Model: Key Terms

Across the fields covered in this book, representative ABMs differ substantially in scope, topic, policy orientation, complexity, and engagement with data. Nonetheless, all these ABMs share a common set of core building blocks. Unpacking these key core elements facilitates comparison among models, replicability, and good design choices.

Building on Hammond (2015), the core elements of an ABM can be conceptualized using the "PARTE" framework, an easily remembered acronym which stands for: properties, actions, rules, time, and environment. The agents in an ABM are defined by the first three elements (properties, actions, and rules cover "who are the agents and what do they do?"), and the context is defined by the remainder (time and environment cover "what is the setting in which the

New Horizons in Modeling and Simulation for Social Epidemiology and Public Health,
First Edition. Daniel Kim.

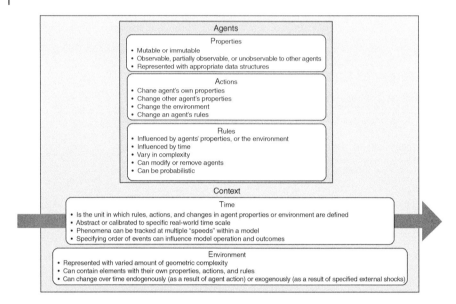

Figure 3.1   The PARTE framework. *Source*: Reproduced from Hammond (2015).

agents do what they do?"). Figure 3.1 illustrates this framework, outlining several of the key choices that a modeler must make when designing an ABM.

Properties define who the agents are – the set of characteristics that differ across individual actors and play an important role in the model. Common agent properties in models focused on the social determinants of health include age, sex, race/ ethnicity, income, education, body mass index, physical activity level, physical and genetic conditions, mental health, and food preferences. The properties of an agent can, for the purposes of the simulation model, be treated as static (i.e. constant over time), playing a role as inputs into some elements of the dynamics. Alternatively, properties can change in value over time either exogenously (e.g. driven by a data table or fixed progression from factors outside the model) or endogenously (because they are altered by the dynamic processes within the model). For example, in a model of diet behavior among adolescents in a particular school classroom, age might be treated as a static variable. In a model simulating early life influences on later health outcomes using cohort data, age might be treated as dynamic but progressing exogenously. Finally, in a model of maternal survival, progression of age might be affected endogenously.

Some properties of an agent may be fully or partially observable to other actors in the model (e.g. the choice of residence is fully observable to others in a segregation model, or body mass index is approximately observable to others in a model of social influence in obesity). Other properties may be unobservable, like genetic polymorphisms or previous smoking history. From an implementation perspective, properties may be stored in the computational model in a variety of data structures reflecting the hypothesized structure of the characteristics – whether Boolean, discrete, continuous, multivariate, etc. Each property of each agent must also be assigned a well-considered initial value, as well as conditions for change, if any.

Actions represent the available set of behaviors for any type of agents. These may be inward facing – changing an agent's own properties (e.g. updating of body mass or age), or outward facing – changing the properties of other agents (e.g. transmitting information), or modifying the environment (e.g. consumption that reduces local availability of an item for other agents). Actions can also potentially change an agent's own rules (e.g. through learning). Each action must have well-defined conditions under which it is triggered (via rules if it is endogenous or via time or environment if exogenous) and well-defined consequences. These triggers and consequences may be deterministic – they occur automatically when a condition is met – or stochastic – they occur with some probability. Actions may not only modify other existing agents – they may also create new agents or remove current ones.

Rules govern the core dynamics of an ABM. They consist of algorithms that define when and why agents perform actions, update properties, and interact with each other and their environment. Given the flexibility of the ABM approach, there can be enormous heterogeneity in rules both within and across models. Rules can range from simple heuristics to full-blown analytical models and can incorporate inputs from within the model (current or past values of own or other's properties), from the environment, and from outside the model boundary (e.g. from data). They can be deterministic or stochastic and interact with time in determining frequency or function.

Time is a core concept for any dynamic simulation model, including an ABM. In most ABMs, time is demarcated in a single discrete fine-grained unit of time – sometimes called a "tick," "iteration," or "round." Action within the model is thus timed in single or multiple iteration intervals – different pieces of the dynamics may move at different speeds but share this common benchmark and are generally expressed in multiples of the finest grained time step. The iteration is an abstract concept, well defined only within the boundary of the model. It can be calibrated in some cases to real-world time periods (e.g. minutes, days, hours, and years) with additional work. Within an ABM, decisions about time can sometimes strongly shape the outcomes, as many ABMs are sensitive to the order in which instructions are followed by the computer.

Environment provides a context in which the agents and their activities unfold. In many ABMs, the environment consists of a spatial geometry of some sort (although this is not required by the technique). Such geometries can range from simple (lattice or torus) to complex (GIS map or network). The environment may contain its own properties, actions, and rules – in some cases functioning as a "sessile" type of agent – or may simply be used to calculate distance or adjacency between agents. Within an ABM, the environment may also change over time endogenously (as a result of agent actions or conditions) or exogenously (to represent known environmental change in the real world or to simulate an exogenous shock to a system). For example, a policy that creates new grocery stores in a food desert is an exogenous change. But if grocery stores open and close in response to agent demand, that is an endogenous change.

This PARTE framework allows explication of the core building blocks for any ABM and comparison among very different specific ABMs. As the descriptions above demonstrate, enormous variability is possible in the specific form each element (P, A, R, T, E) takes. This flexibility is an important part of the power of the ABM approach and also underscores the importance of following best practices in making design and implementation choices (Hammond 2015).

3.2 Steps in Designing and Deploying an Agent-Based Model

The use of ABM within a scientific enterprise generally follows a set of standard steps, covering design, implementation, testing, analysis, and interpretation. These general steps are shared with many other forms of computational modeling but involve particular considerations for ABM as generally practiced in social and health sciences. The summary below describes the basic steps; for more detailed discussion of the associated best practices involved in the use of ABM, see Hammond (2015).

The steps are:

1) Design
    a) problem definition and goal of the model
    b) define model boundaries
    c) operationalize the concepts contained in the model
    d) translate operationalized model into computational code
2) Implementation – testing extreme values and calibration
3) Experimentation – generate hypothetical scenarios to examine with the model
4) Analysis – statistically analyze model outputs and run sensitivity analysis
5) Interpretation – review results in light of research questions (1a) and interpret

The first step, model design, is composed of four parts. *Step 1A*: articulate a clear definition of the specific question(s) the model-based analysis will try to answer, and the goal the model will be designed to serve; this question and goal provide critical guidance for decisions later in the process. *Step 1B*: define a model boundary and initial conceptual design. This includes identifying key concepts or relationships from the literature (initial choices for P, A, and R), along with a clearly defined context for the model (T and E). *Step 1C*: create a detailed model specification, moving from the conceptual design to an operationalized design ready for implementation into computational code. Then, in *Step 1D*, this specification is translated into a computationally functional simulation program, with important best practices for error checking and for ensuring that the elements of the original idea of the model are coded appropriately. The process of computational implementation can sometimes uncover underspecified elements from Step 1C requiring further design work. Also in this step, initial model parameter values are determined.

The next three steps comprise analysis using the ABM model. In *Step 2*, the functioning simulation model is put through a series of testing and calibration exercises. These may include extreme value, boundary adequacy, and face-validity checks, as well as comparison with empirical data. A wide variety of strategies for calibration and validation of agent-based models have been developed over the past five years and are covered in detail elsewhere in both book-length and in summary articles across a number of social science fields (see, for example, Bruch and Atwell 2015; Gallegati et al. 2017; Gatti et al. 2018; Guerini and Moneta 2017; Heard et al. 2015; Heppenstall et al. 2012; Lamperti et al. 2018; Lux and Zwinkels 2018; Marshall and Galea 2015; Nianogo and Arah 2015; Smith et al. 2018; Ward et al. 2016). Findings from this step may lead to revisions of model implementation (Step 1D), specification (Step 1C), or even conceptual design (Step 1B).

In *Step 3*, the analyst designs sets of "experiments" (simulated scenarios and sets of parameterization) that use the model to test hypotheses central to the research focus. Appropriate statistical or other mathematical analysis is conducted on the simulation results as needed to help answer the core research questions, following best practices both for the methodology (ABM) and the field of inquiry (model and audience specific). In *Step 4*, extensive sensitivity analysis is undertaken in which both parameters and assumptions are varied to uncover dependency of results on these choices and to put the Step 3 results into context for interpretation.

In the final step (*Step 5*), findings from experiments and sensitivity analysis (Steps 3 and 4), along with key research questions and goals (Step 1A), are considered to create appropriate interpretations. Results and findings may be visualized or otherwise communicated, and all procedures are documented.

In the process of developing and deploying an ABM, progress through the steps described above is rarely linear – iterative cycles are the norm rather than the exception, especially when one follows the core best practice of beginning with simple models and slowly layering complexity.

Below, we provide a brief history of the use of ABM across fields and its introduction into health science; for more detailed examples of application of ABM in real-world settings, see Chapters 4 and 5.

3.3 History of ABM Application and Categories of ABM Usage

The earliest widespread use of ABM was in biology and social science starting approximately 20 years ago. This work has included study of topics such as:

- evolutionary biology (Axelrod 2004; Hammond and Axelrod 2006; Holland 1992; Nowak 2006; Ohtsuki et al. 2006) and ecology (DeAngelis and Mooij 2005; Heckbert et al. 2010)
- cooperation (Axelrod 1997)
- electoral and bureaucratic dynamics (Bendor and Moe 1985; Bendor et al. 2003; Kollman et al. 1992, 1997; Laver 2005)
- conflict (Bhavnani and Miodownik 2009; Epstein 2002)
- segregation (Bruch and Mare 2006; Schelling 1971; Xie and Zhou 2012). See also Chapter 4.

More recently, ABM use has expanded to education (Maroulis et al. 2014), anthropology (Axtell et al. 2002), economics and finance (Dawid and Neugart 2011; Farmer 2000; Farmer and Foley 2009; LeBaron and Winkler 2008; Tesfatsion and Judd 2006), marketing (North et al. 2010; Rand and Rust 2011), and land use (Berger and Troost 2014; Berger et al. 2007; Brady et al. 2012; Brown et al. 2005a, 2005b; Guzy et al. 2008; Happe et al. 2006, 2008; Heckbert 2011; Magliocca et al. 2014; Sun et al. 2014).

Within the past decade, ABM has seen rapid uptake in public health, initially in the field of epidemiology and control of communicable disease (Burke et al. 2006; Epstein 2004, 2009; Eubank et al. 2004; Ferguson et al. 2006; Germann et al. 2006; Lee et al. 2010; Longini et al. 2005, 2007; Yang et al. 2009). Some of this work will be reviewed in detail in Chapter 5.

More recently, ABM has been used in chronic disease prevention (IOM (The Institute of Medicine) 2010, 2012, 2013; COSSA (Consortium of Social Science Associations) 2014; Hall et al. 2014; Hammond 2009; Hammond and Ornstein 2014; Hammond et al. 2012; Levy et al. 2011; Mabry and Bures 2014; Zhang et al. 2014), social and behavioral aspects of health (Mabry et al. 2013), and health disparities (Kaplan 2017).

The uses of ABM across these many fields vary in purpose and scope. Not all models are (or are intended to be) engaged with empirical data, and not all are directed at policy. The four most common uses of ABM are (i) formulating or testing explanatory hypotheses about (potentially unobservable) mechanisms driving observed patterns in the real world (e.g. formulating and refining hypotheses about etiology), (ii) bridging individual-level assumptions and population-level dynamics, (iii) guiding data collection or empirical analysis by pinpointing especially important gaps or by discovering new questions, and (iv) informing the design or evaluation of interventions (including policy choices).

In the next two chapters, we give a sense of the size of the ABM literature in each of the two areas (social science and public health) and describe in detail specific examples of ABMs used to explicate empirical puzzles. We focus primarily on those models that inform policy choices and encourage the interested reader to return to this chapter to reflect on how the PARTE framework could be applied to parse the models described and on how the models were implemented and communicated, as well as referring back to Chapter 2 to review the key strengths of ABM as a method that are illustrated in many of the examples.

References

Axelrod, R. (1997). *The Complexity of Cooperation: Agent-Based Models of Competition and Collaboration*. NJ: Princeton University Press.

Axelrod, R. (2004). Comparing modeling methodologies. In: *Prepared for CMT International – Project on "Security in Central Asia."*. Ann Arbor, MI: Gerald R. Ford School of Public Policy.

Axtell, R.L., Epstein, J.M., Dean, J.S. et al. (2002). Population growth and collapse in a multiagent model of the Kayenta Anasazi in long house valley. *Proceedings of the National Academy of Sciences of the United States of America* 99: 7275–7279.

Bendor, J. and Moe, T.M. (1985). An adaptive model of bureaucratic politics. *The American Political Science Review* 79 (3): 755–774.

Bendor, J., Diermeier, D., and Ting, M. (2003). A behavioral model of turnout. *American Political Science Review* 97 (2): 261–280.

Berger, T. and Troost, C. (2014). Agent-based modeling of climate adaptation and mitigation options in agriculture. *Journal of Agricultural Economics* 65 (2): 323–348.

Berger, T., Birner, R., McCarthy, N. et al. (2007). Capturing the complexity of water uses and water users within a multi-agent framework. *Water Resources Management* 21 (1): 129–148.

Bhavnani, R. and Miodownik, D. (2009). Ethnic polarization, ethnic salience, and civil war. *Journal of Conflict Resolution* 53 (1): 30–49.

Brady, M., Sahrbacher, C., Kellermann, K. et al. (2012). An agent-based approach to modeling impacts of agricultural policy on land use, biodiversity and ecosystem services. *Landscape Ecology* 27 (9): 1363–1381.

Brown, D.G., Page, S., Riolo, R. et al. (2005a). Path dependence and the validation of agent-based spatial models of land use. *International Journal of Geographical Information Science* 19 (2): 153–174.

Brown, D.G., Riolo, R., Robinson, D.T. et al. (2005b). Spatial process and data models: toward integration of agent-based models and GIS. *Journal of Geographical Systems* 7 (1): 25–47.

Bruch, E.E. and Atwell, J. (2015). Agent-based models in empirical social research. *Sociological Methods & Research* 44 (2): 186–221.

Bruch, E.E. and Mare, R.D. (2006). Neighborhood choice and neighborhood change. *American Journal of Sociology* 112 (3): 667–709.

Burke, D.S., Epstein, J.M., Cummings, D.A. et al. (2006). Individual-based computational modeling of smallpox epidemic control strategies. *Academic Emergency Medicine* 13 (11): 1142–1149.

COSSA (Consortium of Social Science Associations) (2014). OBSSR conference held on complex systems, health disparities and population health: building bridges. www.cossa.org/volume33/OBSSRsystems.pdf (accessed 18 December 2014).

Dawid, H. and Neugart, M. (2011). Agent-based models for economic policy design. *Eastern Economic Journal* 37 (1): 44–50.

DeAngelis, D.L. and Mooij, W.M. (2005). Individual-based modeling of ecological and evolutionary processes. *Annual Review of Ecology, Evolution, and Systematics* 36: 147–168.

Epstein, J.M. (2002). Modeling civil violence: an agent-based computational approach. *Proceedings of the National Academy of Sciences of the United States of America* 99: 7243–7250.

Epstein, J.M. (2004). *Toward a Containment Strategy for Smallpox Bioterror: An Individual-Based Computational Approach*. Washington, DC: Brookings Institution Press.

Epstein, J.M. (2009). Modeling to contain pandemics. *Nature* 460 (7256): 687–687.

Eubank, S., Guclu, H., Kumar, V.A. et al. (2004). Modeling disease outbreaks in realistic urban social networks. *Nature* 429 (6988): 180–184.

Farmer, J.D. (2000). A simple model for the nonequilibrium dynamics and evolution of a financial market. *International Journal of Theoretical and Applied Finance* 3 (3): 425–441.

Farmer, J.D. and Foley, D. (2009). The economy needs agent-based modeling. *Nature* 460 (7256): 685–686.

Ferguson, N.M., Cummings, D.A., Fraser, C. et al. (2006). Strategies for mitigating an influenza pandemic. *Nature* 442 (7101): 448–452.

Gallegati, M., Palestrini, A., and Russo, A. (eds.) (2017). *Introduction to Agent-Based Economics*. New York, NY: Academic Press.

Gatti, D.D., Fagiolo, G., Gallegati, M. et al. (2018). *Agent-Based Models in Economics: A Toolkit*. Cambridge, UK: Cambridge University Press.

Germann, T.C., Kadau, K., Longini, I.M. et al. (2006). Mitigation strategies for pandemic influenza in the United States. *Proceedings of the National Academy of Sciences of the United States of America* 103 (15): 5935–5940.

Guerini, M. and Moneta, A. (2017). A method for agent-based models validation. *Journal of Economic Dynamics and Control* 82: 125–141.

Guzy, M.R., Smith, C.L., Bolte, J.P. et al. (2008). Policy research using agent-based modeling to assess future impacts of urban expansion into farmlands and forests. *Ecology and Society* 13 (1): 37.

Hall, K.D., Hammond, R.A., and Rahmandad, H. (2014). Dynamic interplay among homeostatic, hedonic, and cognitive feedback circuits regulating body weight. *American Journal of Public Health* 104 (7): 1169–1175.

Hammond, R.A. (2009). Complex systems modeling for obesity research. *Preventing Chronic Disease* 6 (3): A97.

Hammond, R.A. (2015). Considerations and best practices in agent-based modeling to inform policy. In: *Assessment of Agent-Based Models to Inform Tobacco Policy* (eds. R. Wallace, A. Geller and V.A. Ogawa), 161–193. Washington, DC: Institute of Medicine, National Academy of Sciences Press.

Hammond, R.A. and Axelrod, R. (2006). Evolution of contingent altruism when cooperation is expensive. *Theoretical Population Biology* 69 (3): 333–338.

Hammond, R.A. and Ornstein, J.T. (2014). A model of social influence on body mass index. *Annals of the New York Academy of Sciences* 1331: 34–42.

Hammond, R.A., Ornstein, J.T., Fellows, L.K. et al. (2012). A model of food reward learning with dynamic reward exposure. *Frontiers in Computational Neuroscience* 6: 82.

Happe, K., Kellermann, K., and Balmann, A. (2006). Agent-based analysis of agricultural policies: An illustration of the agricultural policy simulator agripolis, its adaptation and behavior. *Ecology and Society* 11 (1): 49.

Happe, K., Balmann, A., Kellermann, K. et al. (2008). Does structure matter? The impact of switching the agricultural policy regime on farm structures. *Journal of Economic Behavior & Organization* 67 (2): 431–444.

Heard, D., Dent, G., Schifeling, T. et al. (2015). Agent-based models and microsimulation. *Annual Review of Statistics and Its Applications* 2: 259–272.

Heckbert, S. (2011). Agent-based modeling of emissions trading for coastal landscapes in transition. *Journal of Land Use Science* 6 (2-3): 137–150.

Heckbert, S., Baynes, T., and Reeson, A. (2010). Agent-based modeling in ecological economics. *Annals of the New York Academy of Sciences* 1185 (1): 39–53.

Heppenstall, A.J., Crooks, A.T., See, L.M. et al. (2012). *Agent-Based Models of Geographical Systems*. New York, NY: Springer.

Holland, J. (1992). *Adaptation in Natural and Artificial Systems: An Introductory Analysis with Applications to Biology, Control and Artificial Intelligence*. Cambridge: MIT Press.

IOM (The Institute of Medicine) (2010). *Bridging the Evidence Gap in Obesity Prevention: A Framework to Inform Decision Making* (eds. S.K. Kumanyika, L. Parker and L.J. Sim). Washington, DC: The National Academies Press.

IOM (The Institute of Medicine) (2012). *Accelerating Progress in Obesity Prevention: Solving the Weight of the Nation* (eds. D. Glickman, L. Parker, L.J. Sim, et al.). Washington, DC: The National Academies Press.

IOM (The Institute of Medicine) (2013). *Evaluating Obesity Prevention Efforts: A Plan for Measuring Progress* (eds. L.W. Green, L. Sim and H. Breiner). Washington, DC: The National Academies Press.

Kaplan, G.A. (ed.) (2017). *Growing Inequality: Bridging Complex Systems, Population Health, and Health Disparities.* Washington, DC: Westphalia Press.

Kollman, K., Miller, J.H., and Page, S.E. (1992). Adaptive parties in spatial elections. *American Political Science Review* 86 (4): 929–937.

Kollman, K., Miller, J.H., and Page, S.E. (1997). Political institutions and sorting in a tiebout model. *The American Economic Review* 87 (5): 977–992.

Lamperti, F., Roventini, A., and Sani, A. (2018). Agent-based model calibration using machine learning surrogates. *Journal of Economic Dynamics and Control* 90: 366–389.

Laver, M. (2005). Policy and the dynamics of political competition. *American Political Science Review* 99 (2): 263–281.

LeBaron, B. and Winkler, P. (2008). Agent-based models for economic policy advice [Special issue]. *Journal of Economics and Statistics* 228 (2–3): 141–148.

Lee, B.Y., Brown, S.T., Korch, G. et al. (2010). A computer simulation of vaccine prioritization, allocation, and rationing during the 2009 H1N1 influenza pandemic. *Vaccine* 28 (31): 4875–4879.

Levy, D.T., Mabry, P.L., Wang, Y.C. et al. (2011). Simulation models of obesity: a review of the literature and implications for research and policy. *Obesity Reviews* 12 (5): 378–394.

Longini, I.M. Jr., Halloran, M.E., Nizam, A. et al. (2007). Containing a large bioterrorist smallpox attack: a computer simulation approach. *International Journal of Infectious Diseases* 11 (2): 98–108.

Longini, I.M., Nizam, A., Xu, S. et al. (2005). Containing pandemic influenza at the source. *Science* 309 (5737): 1083–1087.

Lux, T. and Zwinkels, R. (2018). Chapter 8: empirical validation of agent-based models. In: *Handbook of Computational Economics*, vol. 4, 437–488. North Holland: Elsevier.

Mabry, P.L. and Bures, R.M. (2014). Systems science for obesity-related research questions: an introduction to the theme issue. *American Journal of Public Health* 104 (7): 1157–1159.

Mabry, P.L., Milstein, B., Abraido-Lanza, A.F. et al. (2013). Opening a window on systems science research in health promotion and public health. *Health Education and Behavior* 40 (1): 5S–8S.

Magliocca, N.R., Brown, D.G., and Ellis, E.C. (2014). Cross-site comparison of land-use decision-making and its consequences across land systems with a generalized agent-based model. *PLoS One* 9 (1): e86179.

Maroulis, S., Bakshy, E., Gomez, L. et al. (2014). Modeling the transition to public school choice. *Journal of Artificial Societies and Social Simulation* 17 (2): 3.

Marshall, B.D. and Galea, S. (2015). Formalizing the role of agent-based modeling in causal inference and epidemiology. *American Journal of Epidemiology* 181 (2): 92–99.

Nianogo, R.A. and Arah, O.A. (2015). Agent-based modeling of noncommunicable diseases. *American Journal of Public Health* 105 (3): 20–31.

North, M.J., Macal, C.M., Aubin, J.S. et al. (2010). Multiscale agent-based consumer market modeling. *Complexity* 15 (5): 37–47.

Nowak, M.A. (2006). Five rules for the evolution of cooperation. *Science* 314 (5805): 1560–1563.

Ohtsuki, H., Hauert, C., Lieberman, E. et al. (2006). A simple rule for the evolution of cooperation on graphs and social networks. *Nature* 441 (7092): 502–505.

Rand, W. and Rust, R.T. (2011). Agent-based modeling in marketing: guidelines for rigor. *International Journal of Research in Marketing* 28 (3): 181–193.

Schelling, T.C. (1971). Dynamic models of segregation. *Journal of Mathematical Sociology* 1 (2): 143–186.

Smith, N.R., Trauer, J.M., Gambhir, M. et al. (2018). Agent-based models of malaria transmission: a systematic review. *Malaria Journal* 17 (1): 299.

Sun, S., Parker, D.C., Huang, Q. et al. (2014). Market impacts on land-use change: an agent-based experiment. *Annals of the Association of American Geographers* 104 (3): 460–484.

Tesfatsion, L. and Judd, K.L. (2006). *Handbook of Computational Economics: Agent-Based Computational Economics*, vol. 2. Amsterdam: North Holland Publishing Co.

Ward, J.A., Evans, A.J., and Malleson, N.S. (2016). Dynamic calibration of agent-based models using data assimilation. *Royal Society Open Science* 3 (4): 150703.

Xie, Y. and Zhou, X. (2012). Modeling individual-level heterogeneity in racial residential segregation. *Proceedings of the National Academy of Sciences of the United States of America* 109 (29): 11646–11651.

Yang, Y., Sugimoto, J.D., Halloran, M.E. et al. (2009). The transmissibility and control of pandemic influenza a (H1N1) virus. *Science* 326 (5953): 729–733.

Zhang, J., Tong, L., Lamberson, P. et al. (2014). Leveraging social influence to address overweight and obesity using agent-based models: the role of adolescent social networks. *Social Science and Medicine* 125: 203–213.

4

Agent-Based Modeling in the Social Sciences

Joseph T. Ornstein[1] and Ross A. Hammond[1,2,3]

[1] Brown School, Washington University in St. Louis, St. Louis, MO, USA
[2] Center on Social Dynamics & Policy, The Brookings Institution, Washington, DC, USA
[3] The Santa Fe Institute, Santa Fe, NM, USA

4.1 Introduction

In this chapter, we discuss the application of agent-based modeling (ABM) in the social sciences, where the technique has had a longer history than in the health sciences. As case examples, we describe how ABMs helped resolve three significant puzzles in social science: (i) the persistence of racial segregation, (ii) the ubiquity of power laws, and (iii) the depopulation of the Long House Valley by the Ancestral Pueblo Kayenta "Anasazi" people. The first example draws on one of the earliest agent-based models, illustrating how the link between microlevel behavior and macrolevel outcomes is not always intuitive – and how ABM can provide insight into such situations. This example also demonstrates the power of very simple models that do not rely on any large dataset. The second example describes a collection of ABMs that explicate how a ubiquitous statistical pattern can emerge from a few key mechanisms. The final example illustrates how a more complex model, incorporating insights from multiple disciplines, can bring clarity to a very specific and heavily empirical research question. We describe each specific model in some detail, showing how they helped to address the puzzles that motivated the research. For each example, we also give the reader some sense of the related body of empirically oriented ABM work that follows from the model described, using a snowball sample of connected work.

The models described in this chapter provide three important lessons for how modeling can inform social epidemiology and research on the social determinants of health. First, they illustrate the importance of going into a modeling project with an a priori *research question*. A researcher is likely to gain much more clarity if the goal of constructing a model is to answer a specific question, rather than if the goal is vaguely to "model topic X." Research questions help motivate the inevitable assumptions that one must make as a modeler and provide a clear

New Horizons in Modeling and Simulation for Social Epidemiology and Public Health,
First Edition. Daniel Kim.
© 2021 John Wiley & Sons, Inc. Published 2021 by John Wiley & Sons, Inc.

benchmark upon which to compare results (see Chapter 3, step 1a). Second, the example models illustrate the *value of simplicity*. Often the most profound and generalizable insights come from models with very few moving parts, because it is easier to observe what is driving the results, and it is clear whether those results are sensitive to specific assumptions. Finally, we see how agent-based models can foster *interdisciplinary research* by taking insights from multiple disciplines and integrating them into a single theoretical construct.

4.2   Segregation

What is perhaps the first agent-based model in social science was first conceived on a checkerboard. In the late 1960s, the economist Thomas Schelling was flying home from Chicago to Boston. With nothing to read, he began pondering a question. In the 1960s, many US cities had undergone rapid demographic change, as "white flight" resulted in white Americans leaving the urban core for new, auto-dependent suburbs. The result was a striking degree of racial segregation, and most urban neighborhoods were either entirely white or entirely black. Considering these trends, Schelling pondered a simple question: why do groups segregate themselves from one another, and how feasible is it to create racially integrated neighborhoods?

And so, he put together a simple model, doodling with X's and O's on a sheet of graph paper. As soon as he got home, he and his son codified the rules on a checkerboard. The rules are so straightforward that we can play along at home. Consider the checkerboard in Figure 4.1. Suppose that each square is a house, and the checkers represent homeowners. We start by randomly assigning 15 black and 15 white checkers to homes.

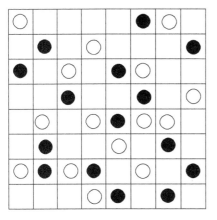

Figure 4.1   Schelling checkerboard (initial state).

Because we have randomly assigned houses, the neighborhood is quite integrated. Checkers typically have both black and white neighbors.

Now, suppose that these checkers (agents) have very simple preferences: they would rather not live in a home where a majority of their neighbors are members of a different race. Crucially, they do not *prefer* segregated neighborhoods; they just prefer not to be in the minority. If an agent is unhappy, they move to a random square. Let us start moving checkers, following this rule:

By the sixth move, we already begin to see segregated neighborhoods forming. There are a few isolated checkers remaining in their original neighborhoods. But as their similar neighbors move out, these checkers become more uncomfortable and are more likely to move themselves. This creates a "tipping point," which eventually results in a completely segregated map. In fact, it only takes eight more moves to reach this final, equilibrium state:[1]

At this point, all of the agents are satisfied with their location, resulting in an *equilibrium* (steady-state) outcome. Even though none of the agents explicitly preferred segregated neighborhoods, collectively they created a situation where integration was impossible.

Why are integrated neighborhoods unstable? In essence, this instability results from a *cascade effect*. When one agent moves to a new home, the decision not only affects themselves, but their neighbors as well. If a white agent moves, it reduces the proportion of white checkers in their original neighborhood, which in turn makes the remaining white checkers more likely to leave. This self-reinforcing feedback loop creates "white flight," making integrated neighborhoods difficult to maintain.

Consider the white checker in Figure 4.1, row 2, column 4 (let us call him Bob). At the beginning of the simulation, Bob is happy. He has one white neighbor and one black neighbor, and he is not a minority in his local neighborhood. However, between Figures 4.2 and 4.3, a sequence of events destabilizes this happy equilibrium. First, a black checker moves to row 4, column 2. This causes the white checker at row 3, column 3 to move away. Now that all of his white neighbors have moved away, Bob is unhappy. In the final round, he moves south, to the newly formed neighborhood of white checkers. Like ripples in a pond, a small perturbation spreads throughout the system, until all of the checkers are sorted by color.

When first introduced to the Schelling (1971) model, many readers are taken aback by its simplicity. The checkerboard layout is quite crude; real neighborhoods are rarely so geometrically orderly. The model does not include any of

---

1 Note that we did not need to choose this particular sequence of moves to generate a segregated outcome. The reader can experiment with different sequences of moves and observe that, in each case, segregation emerges. For particularly interested readers, we suggest exploring the NetLogo library (https://ccl.northwestern.edu/netlogo/index.shtml) where one can find user-friendly computational versions of the models we discuss in this chapter.

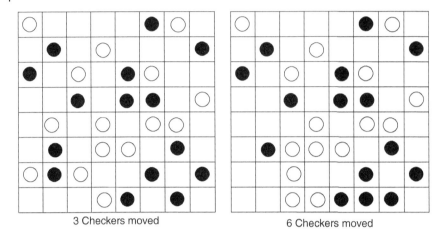

3 Checkers moved   6 Checkers moved

Figure 4.2   Schelling checkerboard (first six moves).

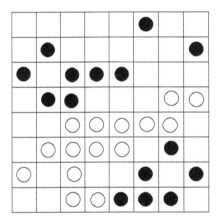

Figure 4.3   Schelling checkerboard (final state).

the vast number of factors that people consider when choosing a neighborhood: home prices, amenities, public schools, commuting costs, etc. It also does not include any of the *explicitly* discriminatory housing policies that historically played a role in creating segregation. These include exclusionary neighborhood covenants (Fischel 2015), race-based discrimination in federal home loan guarantees (Rothstein 2017), real estate steering (Galster 1990; Ondrich et al. 2003), and antidensity zoning ordinances (Rothwell and Massey 2009). Despite these abstractions, the checkerboard model provides an elegant solution to the problem that troubled Thomas Schelling. In this telling of events, white flight and segregation need not be the result of a preference for segregated neighborhoods; segregation can emerge even when no one person desires it. It also suggests that there is an asymmetry between segregation and desegregation. In the model, racial sorting occurs naturally, with very little effort. Integration, however, requires agents to *actively* seek diverse neighbors.[2]

Because the Schelling model is so parsimonious, its empirical performance at *predicting* segregation outcomes is rather mixed. Some authors, such as Card et al. (2008a), find empirical evidence supporting the Schelling model. Examining patterns of racial segregation over three decades at the Census tract level, they find evidence of "tipping points" in the composition of urban neighborhoods. If the minority share of a Census tract exceeded 20% in 1970, that Census tract was much more likely to lose a large share of white households over the subsequent three decades. This is consistent with the dynamics of the Schelling model. On the other hand, Easterly (2009) finds patterns in migration data that are inconsistent with the basic predictions of the Schelling model. Examining the racial composition of US urban neighborhoods between 1970 and 2000, he finds that homogeneous neighborhoods were just as likely to experience "white flight" as integrated neighborhoods, a fact at odds with the cascade effects prediction we describe above.

Given the sheer number of factors that influence neighborhood segregation, it is perhaps unsurprising that the Schelling model alone would not provide good predictions of actual segregation patterns. Nonetheless, it is an excellent example of a model that is *useful* without being empirical. This use of modeling is relatively rare in fields that tend to associate mathematical modeling with statistical methodology. The value of the Schelling model comes not from its fidelity to empirical data but rather from its identifying the sufficient conditions that produce segregation. Even in the absence of discriminatory housing policies, and the absence of economic factors causing people to select racially homogeneous neighborhoods, segregation can still emerge from the microlevel interactions of thousands of independent actors.

Schelling's work changed the direction of the field of social science concerned with understanding and addressing segregation (see the first two lines of Table 4.1), but also both inspired subsequent empirical work and additional agent-based models which together have established firm microfoundations and empirically predictive understandings of segregation patterns in US cities (Table 4.1).

Direct empirical tests of the Schelling model (row i in the table), which predominantly use longitudinal data, surveys, or experiments, find mixed results. Some studies provide evidence of tipping points in residential segregation dynamics by race (Card et al. 2008a,b; Bian et al. 2013) as well as income (Malone 2018); others show that the preferences described in the Schelling model can be observed in real-world surveys (Farley et al. 1978, 1993; Clark 1991; Krysan and Farley 2002). However, other work finds evidence that contradicts the predictions of the

---

2 To see this, consider the neighborhood portrayed in Figure 4.3. If one wanted to reverse the process, producing an integrated neighborhood like in Figure 4.1, it would require agents moving to neighborhoods where they are the minority.

Table 4.1   Selected subsequent papers related to Schelling's original ABM papers.

[A] Total papers that directly cite Schelling (1969)	1354
[B] Total papers that directly cite Schelling (1971)	4038
Among which:	
[i] Direct empirical tests of Schelling's original results	16
[ii] Directly descended ABMs (variations and expansions of Schelling using empirical data)	7
[iii] Other ABMs that cite Schelling's original papers	33

Lines [A] and [B] show counts from a Google Scholar search of papers directly citing each of these original papers. Papers that cite Schelling were briefly reviewed to determine if they contained direct empirical tests of Schelling's original model (row i), new ABMs that were variations or expansions of Schelling incorporating empirical data (row ii), or ABMs on related topics (row iii). This is not intended as a formal literature review or meta-analysis, but instead gives the reader a sense of subsequent work inspired by Schelling's model.

Schelling model, notably Easterly (2009) and Tsvetkova et al. (2016). Some research looks for evidence of the core dynamic at the center of the Schelling findings of the Schelling model in contexts outside neighborhood sorting, including schools (Caetano and Maheshri 2017) and sex segregation in the workforce (England et al. 2007; Pan 2015).

There are a relatively small number of models that both extend the Schelling model of segregation and are grounded in empirical data (row ii). Some of this work supports the idea that the major dynamics of the Schelling model can help explain real-world segregation outcomes. A notable example is Bruch and Mare (2006), who highlight how assumptions about preference functions can change results, and how racial preferences alone are often insufficient to explain segregation outcomes.

Related simulation models that are based on core elements of Schelling's original ABM (row iii) can be found across a variety of fields, including economics (Fagiolo et al. 2007; Pancs and Vriend 2007), sociology (Fossett 2006; Fossett and Dietrich 2009), mathematics (Pollicott and Weiss 2001; Zhang 2004a,b), and physics (Vinković and Kirman 2006; Gauvin et al. 2009). Some of these papers include variations in network structure and agent interaction (Fagiolo et al. 2007; Cortez et al. 2015). Others focus on the sensitivity of segregation outcomes to the addition or variation of key parameters – in addition to racial tolerance and integration preferences (Zhang 2004a; Pancs and Vriend 2007; Radi and Gardini 2015) – including wealth and housing prices (Schnare and MacRae 1978; Zhang 2004b; Bernard and Willer 2007), housing quality preferences (Fossett 2006), location preferences (Chen et al. 2005), city size, shape, and form (Fossett and Dietrich 2009; Spielman and Harrison 2014), neighborhood type (O'Sullivan et al. 2003), and the distance to which agents consider their neighbors (Laurie and Jaggi 2003).

Schelling-type models have also been applied to study segregation in other areas (e.g. school segregation, Stoica and Flache 2014). A large number of papers concur in finding that macroscopic segregation outcomes are generally robust to the inclusion of new parameters or variations in original parameters.

The Schelling model and subsequent literature collectively reveal a deep truth about human society: macrolevel outcomes do not always follow intuitively from the behavior of individual actors. Statistical patterns can emerge that no individual actor or central planner sought out but that instead emerge from the decentralized interactions of individual actors. This idea, which is at the core of the ABM approach, is also vividly illustrated in our next case example.

4.3   Power Laws

In 1896, the Italian economist Vilfredo Pareto made a striking discovery. Studying public records in Italy, he found that land ownership was highly skewed toward the wealthy. A small share of landowners – roughly 20% – owned nearly 80% of the land. Meanwhile, the remaining 80% of the population owned only 20% of the land. This "80-20 rule" was one of the first rigorous quantitative studies on the nature of economic inequality (Pareto 1896). And in over a century since that initial discovery, the same pattern was rediscovered in country after country, year after year. It is such a pervasive empirical regularity that scholars have dubbed it the "Pareto Distribution." And what is particularly remarkable is that this distribution appears not only in dusty old ledgers of Italian landholdings but across a vast array of datasets in the social sciences.

Figure 4.4 illustrates the incredible breadth of topics where Pareto distributions – also called *power laws* – appear. For example, US firm sizes are power law distributed: over 80% of US workers are employed at only 10% of the firms (Axtell 2001). City sizes are power law distributed as well: 20% of US cities have 87% of the population (Gabaix 1999). The phenomenon appears outside of economics too. For instance, interstate wars are power law distributed in their intensity and timing (Clauset 2018). By some estimates, 10% of the wars since 1817 were responsible for 94% of battle deaths (Richardson 1948; Cederman 2003). The frequency of word usage in the literature also follows a power law. Of the top 10 000 words in the corpus of books digitized by Project Gutenberg, 20% were used 86% of the time (Zipf 1949).[3]

---

3 Mathematically, the Pareto distribution follows the following density function: px = Cx-α. In several of these cases, the distribution is actually a special case of the Pareto distribution called a *Zipf distribution*. A Zipf distribution describes a power law where $\alpha = 1$. This implies that doubling the magnitude of an event cuts the frequency of observations in half.

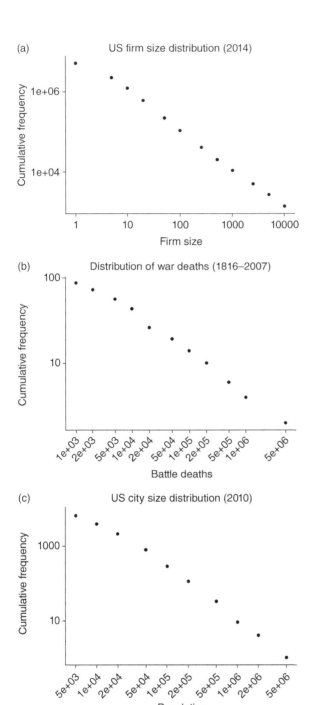

Figure 4.4   Power law phenomena crop up throughout the social sciences: (a) US firm sizes. (b) Battle deaths by war (1816–2007). (c) US city populations (2010). (d) Word usage in English language books. (e) The distribution of Twitter followers among popular accounts. Note the statistical signature of power law distributions: when plotted on log axes, we observe a downward sloping line. Doubling the variable on the x-axis is associated with a proportional decrease in frequency.

(d)

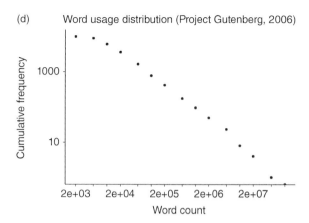

(e)

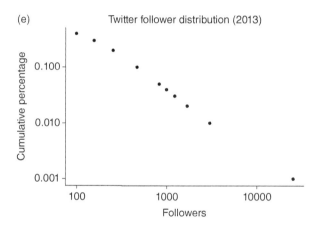

Figure 4.4 (Continued)

There are several important features of power law distributions. The first is that they exhibit extremely *long tails*. A small number of wars account for the preponderance of war deaths. A small number of firms employ the majority of workers. The second feature of power laws is that they are *self-similar*. Not only is a power law distribution highly skewed toward the wealthy, but it is also skewed *among the wealthy*. If one were to take just the wealthiest 20% of US citizens, the distribution of wealth within that subset would *also* be power law distributed.

The ubiquity of power laws across so many disparate fields cries out for an explanation. Is there some universal process that underlies all of these seemingly unrelated topics?

Early attempts to explain the phenomenon were primarily statistical. Simon (1955), for instance, demonstrated that a process of *preferential attachment* could generate power law distributions. Suppose that you have 10 urns and 1000 pebbles.

One by one, you take each pebble and place it in one of the urns, choosing an urn with a probability proportional to the number of pebbles that it already contains. At the beginning of the process, you are equally likely to choose each urn. But as time goes on, one urn will begin to accumulate more pebbles than the others, making you more likely to add pebbles to that urn. And so the rich get richer, and pebbles begin to concentrate in just a few urns. This process gives rise to power laws.

This sort of statistical explanation provides an important first step toward understanding why power laws are so ubiquitous. For example, if large cities are more attractive to immigrants than small cities, then over time, city sizes will converge to a power law distribution. This, however, is not a complete explanation because it simply pushes the question back one level. Why do large cities attract the most migrants? Why would large wars be more likely to escalate, increasing the death toll? What makes large firms better able to attract new employees? With the advent of computational agent-based models, investigating the *mechanisms* underlying these statistical processes became feasible.

In the early 1990s, Josh Epstein and Robert Axtell built an agent-based model of a simple farming economy called Sugarscape (Epstein and Axtell 1996). Like the Schelling model we discussed above, it takes place on a grid of cells. Each cell contains some quantity of sugar, which can be harvested by agents. Agents require sugar to live, and each period they consume some amount of sugar equal to their metabolism. The landscape regenerates over time, as sugar regrows following a harvest.

The behavior of the Sugarscape agents is very straightforward, and they are not particularly rational or forward-thinking. Agents move to a neighboring cell if it is empty and it has more sugar than the cell they currently live on. They save sugar if they harvest more than their metabolic rate, and once they accumulate a large enough sugar surplus, they can spend it to produce offspring.

Epstein and Axtell set up their computational agents with these simple rules and tracked the amount of sugar accumulated by every agent over time. The Sugarscape agents quickly (within a generation or two) converge on the regularity originally observed by Pareto. Wealth naturally gravitates toward a power law distribution, where the wealthiest sugar harvesters accumulate many orders of magnitude more sugar than the poorest.

Following Sugarscape, a flowering of agent-based models emerged to explain power laws in other contexts. Axtell (1999) models the evolution of firm sizes, capturing two competing forces that influence the creation and growth of firms. First, there are economies of scale. Individual agents want to increase their income, and one strategy for doing so is to team up with other agents to create firms. By working together, larger teams produce a surplus beyond what an individual is capable of producing; however, there is also a competing force that limits the size of firms.[4] As firms get too large, they suffer from a free-rider problem. In small firms, it is obvious who is working hard and how much they contribute to the firm's success. But in larger firms, this becomes more and more difficult. As a result, agents in large firms have an incentive to shirk responsibility, which counteracts the efficiency that comes from size. Axtell demonstrates that these two conditions are jointly sufficient to produce power law distributions of firms.

What about the power law distribution of wars? Decades after Richardson (1948) first noted the long-tailed distribution of war deaths, no one had put forward a satisfactory explanation of the phenomenon. Cederman (2003) constructs an agent-based model of nations competing for territory and shows that a power law distribution of war severity can emerge through the interaction of two simple rules. First, the technology of warfare must exhibit a "loss-of-strength gradient" such that a nation must expend more resources to wage war at great distances from their capital city. Second, larger nations are able to extract resources from their territory, which can then be used to wage war for more territory. These two conditions are strikingly similar to the conditions in Axtell's firm size model: the economies of scale in resource extraction push the simulated nations to grow and accumulate territory, while the loss-of-strength gradient puts a limit on how large they are able to become. Over the course of the simulation, the number of simulated nations declines as most are conquered by their neighbors. This historical trajectory in the model matches the actual historical trajectory of European states quite well, which went from over 500 states in the seventeenth century to less than 20 in the twentieth century. And as the nations become larger and less numerous, the intensity of warfare increases. By the end of each simulation, the distribution of resources expended in each war is perfectly described by a power law.

By unpacking in some detail a set of mechanistic processes by which power laws emerge naturally from the decentralized interactions of individuals, their ubiquity as a statistical pattern becomes much less of a puzzle (and a much more practically useful signal of dynamics for a scientist or policymaker). Our third example is the most empirically detailed (and complex) of the agent-based models described here but also has the most concrete focus – an ancient civilization in a real-world place in the American Southwest.

---

4 If there were no such competing force, then all the agents would join together to create a "superfirm," and there would be no small firms at all.

4.4   The Anasazi

For over three millennia, a group of Ancestral Pueblo Native Americans inhabited the Long House Valley region of Arizona (Figure 4.5); at the time of the publication of the paper we will be discussing here, this group was generally referred to as the Anasazi, so we use this term for parsimony though today they are more frequently referred to as the Kayenta. Archaeological evidence suggests that at its peak in the thirteenth century AD, there were over 200 households living in the 96-km^2 valley. They created distinctive black-on-white painted ceramics and gray-textured cooking pottery and built their homes and structures using sophisticated stone masonry.

And then, within the course of a few years, the Anasazi left Long House Valley. After 1275 AD, the archaeological record ceases, and there are no signs of settlement in the valley until the modern era.[5]

For decades, anthropologists debated the causes of this abandonment. Were the Kayenta Anasazi killed off by famine? Drought? Warfare? Or did they simply abandon the valley? And if so, what spurred their migration after such a long period of stability?

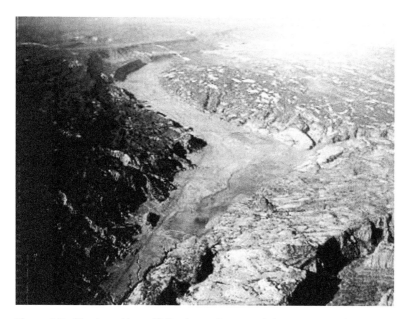

Figure 4.5   The Long House Valley in northeastern Arizona, present day.

---

5 For a more in-depth recounting of this history, see Dan Bailey's 2011 *Scientific American* article, "In search of the origins of warfare in the American Southwest," and on the development of the agent-based model, see Johnathan Rauch's 2002 *Atlantic* article "Seeing Around Corners."

This sort of research may seem to be an unlikely candidate for ABM. How can a computer simulation yield insight into a centuries-old mystery? Anthropologists typically rely on archaeological evidence and historical records to resolve these sorts of disputes. Nevertheless, the question of what became of the Anasazi proved to be a perfect subject for ABM. One great advantage of the method is that it can incorporate large amounts of data from very disparate sources. And over several decades, anthropologists and environmental scientists had accumulated an impressive array of data on the ancient Long House Valley. These included centuries of tree ring data, recording the ebbs and flows of alluvial groundwater. They also included detailed counts and locations of Anasazi households for the five centuries between 800 and 1300 AD. And, importantly, the case in question occurred in a relatively remote geographic area, so it can be considered in isolation from what was happening in the rest of the American Southwest at that time.

And so, in late 2001, an interdisciplinary team of computational modelers, archaeologists, anthropologists, and tree ring experts set out to construct an agent-based model of population growth and decline in the Long House Valley (Axtell et al. 2002). They had a very specific question in mind: could environmental factors alone have forced the Anasazi to abandon the Long House Valley?

As a first step, the modeling team combined historical records of drought severity (Palmer 1965) with a statistical analysis of drought and crop yields (Van West 1994) to create a dynamic landscape of annual potential maize production between the year 800 and 1300 AD. Figure 4.6 displays a snapshot of that landscape in two representative years.

Once the environment was created, they populated the model with artificial Anasazi agents. These agents follow simple rules, derived from ethnographic studies of historic Pueblo peoples. Each year, they require a certain number of calories to survive and to produce offspring. New households are formed in unoccupied arable land if there is a calorie surplus, and households are removed when there is not enough nearby arable land to support them. Over time, the ABM reproduced observed settlement patterns in the Long House Valley; agents locate in areas of fruitful soil, as did the actual Anasazi.

The ABM revealed an important fact: a multidecade drought beginning in the 1250s decreased the carrying capacity of the Long House Valley, but it likely did *not* render the valley uninhabitable. The simulation suggests that the valley could have supported several dozen Anasazi households well into the fourteenth century. Instead, archaeological records suggest that the population collapsed. Taken together, the implication of these findings is that the Anasazi abandoned the valley willingly, as a result of cultural rather than environmental forces.

Additional anthropological evidence eventually came to light regarding the fate of the Kayenta Anasazi. They did not die out but instead migrated to other areas of the southwest. Evidence from mitochondrial DNA suggests that their

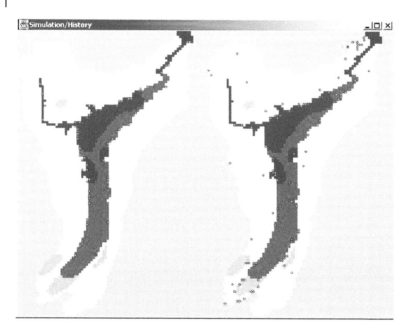

Figure 4.6   Dynamic landscape of potential maize production in Long House Valley.

Table 4.2   Selected subsequent papers related to Axtell et al.'s original ABM paper.

[A] Direct cite to Axtell et al. (2002)	369
[i] Empirical papers that cite Axtell et al. (2002)	6
[ii] Related subsequent empirical ABMs that cite Axtell et al. (2002)	31

Line [A] shows count from a Google Scholar search of papers directly citing this 2002 paper. These were briefly reviewed to determine if they contained direct empirical engagement with Axtell et al.'s original model (row i), or new ABMs that were related to this original model and incorporated empirical data (row ii). This is not intended as a formal literature review or meta-analysis, but instead gives the reader a sense of subsequent work inspired by the Axtell et al. (2002) paper.

descendants would, in subsequent centuries, become the modern-day Zuni and Hopi (Carlyle et al. 2000).

Like the Schelling paper described above, the Axtell et al. (2002) paper is widely cited (Table 4.2, line A) and led to a number of subsequent empirical papers (Table 4.2, line i) and related agent-based models (Table 4.2, line ii). Several of these attempt to directly recreate the model from the seminal paper – or aspects of the model – in order to test the robustness of its conclusions to variations in key parameters (Janssen 2009; Gunaratne and Garibay 2017) or use it as case study to

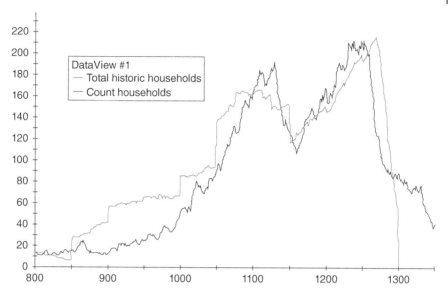

Figure 4.7   Actual and simulated population of Long House Valley between 800 and 1300 AD.

explore the application of a computer algorithm to improve the calibration process (Stonedahl and Wilensky 2010) (Figure 4.7).

A number of related models of socioecological systems, which cite the original Axtell et al. piece as inspiration, involve the interaction between human populations and the environment and (in the spirit of Axtell et al. 2002) rely heavily on real-world evidence for parameterization and calibration. Many of these models also attempt to answer open questions difficult to resolve via traditional approaches. One set of papers is focused on farmer–herder populations from prehistoric times (Macmillan and Huang 2008; Wainwright 2008; Rouleau et al. 2009; Barton et al. 2010; Flores et al. 2011; Gabler 2012; Machálek et al. 2012; Callegari et al. 2013; Smaldino et al. 2013; Baum 2014; Chliaoutakis and Chalkiadakis 2016); others focus primarily on human migration in a similar era of history (Rouly and Crooks 2010; Pardo-Gordó et al. 2017). A second set of papers primarily addresses questions in the anthropological record regarding resource exchange or conflict (Flores and Bologna 2013; Duering and Wahl 2014; Froese et al. 2014; Ortega et al. 2014, 2016; Olševičová et al. 2015; Roman et al. 2017).

Within the archaeological and ecological science communities, several new lines of research using ABM have arisen since the Axtell et al. (2002) paper. Among the most prominent of these is the Village Ecodynamics Project (Crabtree et al. 2017; Kohler et al. 2008, 2012; Kohler and Varien 2012), focused on the Pueblo Indian population in Southwestern Colorado, which includes study of agent relocation behavior as well as exchange of food between households. Other work explores the response of human actors to environmental change in various settings using ABM (Barton 2014; Heckbert et al. 2016; Millán et al. 2016; Barton et al. 2015; Perry and O'Sullivan 2018; Contreras et al. 2019; Rogers and Cegielski 2017). An additional important field of study uses ABM to explore the likely effects of current-day climate change and drought on the displacement and adaptation of modern societies (Berman et al. 2004; Bithell and Brasington 2009; Guedes et al. 2016).

4.5 Conclusions

ABM has been used in social sciences for several decades and (as the examples below illustrate) has in many cases been able to provide explanatory and even predictive power empirically. This success – along with specific lessons learned and concrete empirical insights on relevant topics like segregation – forms an important source of inspiration for the use of ABM in understanding the social determinants of health. In the next chapter, we review early important examples of the use of ABM within the public health arena.

References

Axtell, R. (1999). The emergence of firms in a population of agents: local increasing returns, unstable Nash equilibria, and power law size distributions. *Center on Social and Economic Dynamics Working Paper* 3: 1–108.

Axtell, R.L. (2001). Zipf distribution of US firm sizes. *Science* 293 (5536): 1818–1820.

Axtell, R.L., Epstein, J.M., Dean, J.S. et al. (2002). Population growth and collapse in a multiagent model of the Kayenta Anasazi in Long House Valley. *Proceedings of the National Academy of Sciences of the United States of America* 99: 7275–7279.

Barton, C.M. (2014). Complexity, social complexity, and modeling. *Journal of Archaeological Method and Theory* 21 (2): 306–324.

Barton, C.M., Ullah, I., and Mitasova, H. (2010). Computational modeling and Neolithic socioecological dynamics: a case study from southwest Asia. *American Antiquity* 75 (2): 364–386.

Barton, C.M., Ullah, I., and Heimsath, A. (2015). How to make a barranco: modeling erosion and landscape use in Mediterranean landscapes. *Land* 4 (3): 578–606.

Baum, T.G. (2014). Models of wetland settlement and associated land use in South-West Germany during the fourth millennium b.c. *Vegetation History and Archaeobotany* 23 (1): 67–80.

Berman, M., Nicolson, C., Kofinas, G. et al. (2004). Adaptation and sustainability in a small arctic community: results of an agent-based simulation model. *Arctic* 57 (4): 401–414.

Bernard, S. and Willer, R. (2007). A wealth and status-based model of residential segregation. *Mathematical Sociology* 31 (2): 149–174.

Bian, X., Brastow, R., Waller, B.D. et al. (2013). Neighborhood tipping and sorting dynamics in real estate: evidence from the virginia sex offender registry. SSRN: dx.doi.org/10.2139/ssrn.2338223

Bithell, M. and Brasington, J. (2009). Coupling agent-based models of subsistence farming with individual-based forest models and dynamic models of water distribution. *Environmental Modelling and Software* 24 (2): 173–190.

Bruch, E.E. and Mare, R.D. (2006). Neighborhood choice and neighborhood change. *American Journal of Sociology* 112 (3): 667–709.

Caetano, G. and Maheshri, V. (2017). School segregation and the identification of tipping behavior. *Journal of Public Economics* 148: 115–135.

Callegari, S., Weissmann, J.D., Tkachenko, N. et al. (2013). An agent-based model of human dispersals at a global scale. *Advances in Complex Systems* 16 (4–5): 1350023.

Card, D., Mas, A., and Rothstein, J. (2008a). Tipping and the dynamics of segregation. *The Quarterly Journal of Economics* 123 (1): 177–218.

Card, D., Mas, A., and Rothstein, J. (2008b). *Are Mixed Neighborhoods Always Unstable? Two-Sided and One-Sided Tipping* (No. w14470). National Bureau of Economic Research.

Carlyle, S.W., Parr, R.L., Hayes, M.G. et al. (2000). Context of maternal lineages in the greater southwest. *American Journal of Physical Anthropology* 113 (1): 85–101.

Cederman, L. (2003). Modeling the size of wars: from billiard balls to sandpiles. *The American Political Science Review* 97 (1): 135–150.

Chen, K., Irwin, E.G., Jayaprakash, C. et al. (2005). The emergence of racial segregation in an agent-based model of residential segregation location: the role of competing preferences. *Computational and Mathematical Organization Theory* 11 (4): 333–338.

Chliaoutakis, A. and Chalkiadakis, G. (2016). Agent-based modeling of ancient societies and their organization structure. *Autonomous Agents and Multi-Agent Systems* 30 (6): 1072–1116.

Clark, W.A. (1991). Residential preferences and neighborhood racial segregation: a test of the Schelling segregation model. *Demography* 28 (1): 1–19.

Clauset, A. (2018). Trends and fluctuations in the severity of interstate wars. *Science Advances* 4 (2): eaao3580.

Contreras, D.A., Bondeau, A., Guiot, J. et al. (2019). From paleoclimate variables to prehistoric agriculture: using a process-based agro-ecosystem model to simulate the impacts of Holocene climate change on potential agricultural productivity in Provence, France. *Quaternary International* 501: 303–316.

Cortez, V., Medina, P., Goles, E. et al. (2015). Attractors, statistics and fluctuations of the dynamics of the Schelling's model for social segregation. *The European Physical Journal B* 88 (1): 25.

Crabtree, S.A., Bocinsky, R.K., Hooper, P.L. et al. (2017). How to make a polity in the central mesa verde region. *American Antiquity* 82 (1): 71–95.

Duering, A. and Wahl, J. (2014). A massacred village community? Agent-based modelling sheds new light on the demography of the Neolithic mass grave of Talheim. *Anthropologischer Anzeiger* 71 (4): 447–468.

Easterly, W. (2009). Empirics of strategic interdependence: the case of the racial tipping point. *The BE Journal of Macroeconomics* 9 (1): 1–35.

England, P., Allison, P., Li, S. et al. (2007). Why are some academic fields tipping toward female? The sex composition of US fields of doctoral degree receipt, 1971–2002. *Sociology of Education* 80 (1): 23–42.

Epstein, J.M. and Axtell, R. (1996). *Growing Artificial Societies: Social Science from the Bottom Up*. Washington, DC/Cambridge, MA: Brookings Institution Press.

Fagiolo, G., Valente, M., and Vriend, N.J. (2007). Segregation in networks. *Journal of Economic Behavior and Organization* 64 (3–4): 316–336.

Farley, R., Schuman, H., Bianchi, S. et al. (1978). "Chocolate city, vanilla suburbs:" will the trend toward racially separate communities continue? *Social Science Research* 7 (4): 319–344.

Farley, R., Steeh, C., Jackson, T. et al. (1993). Continued racial residential segregation in Detroit: "chocolate city, vanilla suburbs" revisited. *Journal of Housing Research* 4 (1): 1–38.

Fischel, W.A. (2015). *Zoning Rules! The Economics of Land Use Regulation*. Cambridge: Lincoln Institute of Land Policy.

Flores, J.C. and Bologna, M. (2013). Troy: a simple nonlinear mathematical perspective. *Physica A: Statistical Mechanics and Its Applications* 392 (19): 4683–4687.

Flores, J.C., Bologna, M., and Urzagasti, D. (2011). A mathematical model for the Andean Tiwanaku civilization collapse: climate variations. *Journal of Theoretical Biology* 291: 29–32.

Fossett, M. (2006). Ethnic preferences, social distance dynamics, and residential segregation: theoretical explorations using simulation analysis. *Journal of Mathematical Sociology* 30 (3–4): 185–273.

Fossett, M. and Dietrich, D.R. (2009). Effects of city size, shape, and form, and neighborhood size and shape in agent-based models of residential segregation: are Schelling-style preference effects robust? *Environment and Planning B: Planning and Design* 36 (1): 149–169.

Froese, T., Gershenson, C., and Manzanilla, L.R. (2014). Can government be self-organized? A mathematical model of the collective social organization of ancient Teotihuacan, Central Mexico. *PloS One* 9 (10): e109966.

Gabaix, X. (1999). Zipf's law for cities: an explanation. *The Quarterly Journal of Economics* 114 (3): 739–767.

Gabler, B.M. (2012). Modeling livestock's contribution to the duration of the village farming lifeway in pre-state societies. *Journal of Ecological Anthropology* 15 (1): 5–21.

Galster, G. (1990). Racial steering by real estate agents: mechanisms and motives. *The Review of Black Political Economy* 19 (1): 39–63.

Gauvin, L., Vannimenus, J., and Nadal, J.P. (2009). Phase diagram of a Schelling segregation model. *The European Physical Journal B* 70 (2): 293–304.

Guedes, J.A., Crabtree, S.A., Bocinsky, R.K. et al. (2016). Twenty-first century approaches to ancient problems: climate and society. *Proceedings of the National Academy of Sciences of the United States of America* 113 (51): 14483–14491.

Gunaratne, C. and Garibay, I. (2017). Alternate social theory discovery using genetic programming: towards better understanding the artificial Anasazi. Proceedings of GECCO '17, Berlin, Germany (15–19 July 2017). Association for Computing Machinery.

Heckbert, S., Isendahl, C., Gunn, J.D. et al. (2016). Growing the ancient Maya social-ecological system from the bottom up. In: *The Oxford Handbook of Historical Ecology and Applied Archaeology* (eds. C. Isendahl and D. Stump). Oxford University Press.

Janssen, M.A. (2009). Understanding artificial Anasazi. *Journal of Artificial Societies and Social Simulation* 12 (4): 13.

Kohler, T.A. and Varien, M.D. (2012). *Emergence and Collapse of Early Villages*. Berkeley, CA: University of California Press.

Kohler, T.A., Varien, M.D., Wright, A.M. et al. (2008). Mesa verde migrations: new archaeological research and computer simulation suggest why ancestral Puebloans deserted the northern Southwest United States. *American Scientist* 96 (2): 146–153.

Kohler, T.A., Bocinsky, R.K., Cockburn, D. et al. (2012). Modelling prehispanic Pueblo societies in their ecosystems. *Ecological Modelling* 241: 30–41.

Krysan, M. and Farley, R. (2002). The residential preferences of blacks: do they explain persistent segregation? *Social Forces* 80 (3): 937–980.

Laurie, A.J. and Jaggi, N.K. (2003). Role of 'vision' in neighbourhood racial segregation: a variant of the Schelling segregation model. *Urban Studies* 40 (13): 2687–2704.

Machálek, T., Olševičová, K. and Cimler, R. (2012). Modelling population dynamics for archaeological simulations. Proceedings of 30th International Conference Mathematical Methods in Economics, Silesian University School of Business Administration, Karviná, Czech Republic (11–13 September 2012).

Macmillan, W. and Huang, H.Q. (2008). An agent-based simulation model of a primitive agricultural society. *Geoforum* 39 (2): 643–658.

Malone, T. (2018). There goes the neighborhood: does tipping exist amongst income groups? SSRN: dx.doi.org/10.2139/ssrn.3045793

Millán, E.N., Goirán, S., Forconesi, L. et al. (2016). Monte Carlo model framework to simulate settlement dynamics. *Ecological Informatics* 36: 135–144.

O'Sullivan, D., MacGill, J. and Yu, C. (2003). Agent-based residential segregation: a hierarchically structured spatial model. *Proceedings of agent 2003 conference on challenges in social simulation*, (2–4 October 2003). Chicago, IL: University of Chicago.

Olševičová, K., Procházka, J. and Danielisová, A. (2015). Reconstruction of prehistoric settlement network using agent-based model in NetLogo. *International Conference on Practical Applications of Agents and Multi-Agent Systems*, Salamanca, Spain (3–4 June 2015). Springer.

Ondrich, J., Ross, S., and Yinger, J. (2003). Now you see it, now you don't: why do real estate agents withhold available houses from black customers? *Review of Economics and Statistics* 85 (4): 854–873.

Ortega, D., Ibañez, J.J., Khalidi, L. et al. (2014). Towards a multi-agent-based modelling of obsidian exchange in the Neolithic Near East. *Journal of Archaeological Method and Theory* 21 (2): 461–485.

Ortega, D., Ibáñez, J.J., Campos, D. et al. (2016). Systems of interaction between the first sedentary villages in the near east exposed using agent-based modelling of Obsidian exchange. *Systems* 4 (2): 18.

Palmer, W.C. (1965). Meteorological drought. Research Paper 45. United States Weather Bureau.

Pan, J. (2015). Gender segregation in occupations: the role of tipping and social interactions. *Journal of Labor Economics* 33 (2): 365–408.

Pancs, R. and Vriend, N.J. (2007). Schelling's spatial proximity model of segregation revisited. *Journal of Public Economics* 91 (1–2): 1–24.

Pardo-Gordó, S., Bergin, S.M., Aubán, J.B. et al. (2017). Alternative stories of agricultural origins: the Neolithic spread in the Iberian Peninsula. In: *Times of Neolithic Transition along the Western Mediterranean* (eds. O. García-Puchol and D.C. Salazar-García), 101–131. Cham: Springer.

Pareto, V. (1896). *Cours d'Économie Politique*. Lausanne: Professé a l'Université de Lausanne.

Perry, G.L. and O'Sullivan, D. (2018). Identifying narrative descriptions in agent-based models representing past human-environment interactions. *Journal of Archaeological Method and Theory* 25 (3): 795–817.

Pollicott, M. and Weiss, H. (2001). The dynamics of Schelling-type segregation models and a nonlinear graph Laplacian variational problem. *Advances in Applied Mathematics* 27 (1): 17–40.

Radi, D. and Gardini, L. (2015). Entry limitations and heterogeneous tolerances in a Schelling-like segregation model. *Chaos, Solitons and Fractals* 79: 130–144.

Richardson, L.F. (1948). Variation of the frequency of fatal quarrels with magnitude. *American Statistical Association* 43: 523–546.

Rogers, J.D. and Cegielski, W.H. (2017). Opinion: building a better past with the help of agent-based modeling. *Proceedings of the National Academy of Sciences of the United States of America* 114 (49): 12841–12844.

Roman, S., Bullock, S., and Brede, M. (2017). Coupled societies are more robust against collapse: a hypothetical look at Easter Island. *Ecological Economics* 132: 264–278.

Rothstein, R. (2017). *The Color of Law: A Forgotten History of How Our Government Segregated America*. New York; London: Liveright Publishing.

Rothwell, J. and Massey, D.S. (2009). The effect of density zoning on racial segregation in u.s. urban areas. *Urban Affairs Review* 44 (6): 779–806.

Rouleau, M., Coletti, M., Bassett, J.K. et al. (2009). Conflict in complex socio-natural systems: using agent-based modeling to understand the behavioral roots of social unrest within the Mandera Triangle. *Proceedings of the Human Behavior-Computational Modeling and Interoperability Conference 2009 HB-CMI-09*, (22–24 June 2009). Oak Ridge, Tennessee: Joint Institute for Computational Science, Oak Ridge National Laboratory.

Rouly, O.C. and Crooks, A. (2010). A prototype, multi-agent system for the study of the Peopling of the Western Hemisphere. *Proceedings of the 3rd World Congress on Social Simulation: Scientific Advances in Understanding Societal Processes and Dynamics*, (September 2010). Kassel, Germany: University of Kassel.

Schelling, T.C. (1969). Models of segregation. *The American Economic Review* 59 (2): 488–493.

Schelling, T.C. (1971). Dynamic models of segregation. *Journal of Mathematical Sociology* 1: 143–186.

Schnare, A.B. and MacRae, C.D. (1978). The dynamics of neighbourhood change. *Urban Studies* 15 (3): 327–331.

Simon, H.A. (1955). On a class of skew distribution functions. *Biometrika* 42 (3): 425–440.

Smaldino, P.E., Newson, L., Schank, J.C. et al. (2013). Simulating the evolution of the human family: cooperative breeding increases in harsh environments. *PLoS One* 8 (11).

Spielman, S. and Harrison, P. (2014). The coevolution of residential segregation and the built environment at the turn of the 20th century: a Schelling model. *Transactions in GIS* 18 (1): 25–45.

Stoica, V.I. and Flache, A. (2014). From Schelling to schools: a comparison of a model of residential segregation with a model of school segregation. *Journal of Artificial Societies and Social Simulation* 17 (1): 5.

Stonedahl, F. and Wilensky, U. (2010). Evolutionary robustness checking in the artificial Anasazi model. AAAI Fall Symposium: Complex Adaptive Systems (120–129).

Tsvetkova, M., Nilsson, O., Öhman, C. et al. (2016). An experimental study of segregation mechanisms. *EPJ Data Science* 5 (1): 4.

Van West, C.R. (1994). *Modeling Prehistoric Agricultural Productivity in Southwestern Colorado: A GIS Approach*. Pullman: Washington State University.

Vinković, D. and Kirman, A. (2006). A physical analogue of the Schelling model. *Proceedings of the National Academy of Sciences of the United States of America* 103 (51): 19261–19265.

Wainwright, J. (2008). Can modelling enable us to understand the role of humans in landscape evolution? *Geoforum* 39 (2): 659–674.

Zhang, J. (2004a). A dynamic model of residential segregation. *Journal of Mathematical Sociology* 28 (3): 147–170.

Zhang, J. (2004b). Residential segregation in an all-integrationist world. *Journal of Economic Behavior and Organization* 54 (4): 533–550.

Zipf, G.K. (1949). *Human Behaviour and the Principle of Least-Effort*. Cambridge, MA: Addison-Wesley.

5

Agent-Based Modeling in Public Health

Joseph T. Ornstein[1] and Ross A. Hammond[1,2,3]

[1] Brown School, Washington University in St. Louis, St. Louis, MO, USA
[2] Center on Social Dynamics & Policy, The Brookings Institution, Washington, DC, USA
[3] The Santa Fe Institute, Santa Fe, NM, USA

5.1   Introduction

In the past decade, there has been an explosion of research applying agent-based modeling (ABM) to the study of public health. In this chapter, we present a formal literature search, giving the reader a sense of the scale and scope of work in this area to date. We then select a number of exemplary papers in the field for more detailed review. In particular, we discuss agent-based models in three subfields where their use has been most prevalent in public health to date: infectious disease, obesity, and tobacco control.

For each set of topics, we focus on illustrative articles that satisfy three conditions. First, each article presents the results of an original agent-based model, demonstrating the added value of such computational modeling for addressing research questions in public health. Second, they are all empirically grounded in some way, either calibrating parameters based on empirical analysis of data or comparing outputs against observed patterns. The most fully developed models produce true out-of-sample predictions, demonstrating that the models can generate patterns observed in a dataset that was not used to calibrate the inputs. Finally, these papers leverage a core strength of agent-based models – their ability to represent social interactions – and use this strength to explore the *social drivers* of infectious disease, obesity, and tobacco use.

5.2   Scale of ABM Usage in Public Health

To document the scale of ABM usage in public health to date, we performed formal literature searches in each of the three distinct topic areas using two databases: Scopus and Web of Science Core Collection Database. We provide the full

New Horizons in Modeling and Simulation for Social Epidemiology and Public Health,
First Edition. Daniel Kim.

Table 5.1 Number of hits from the literature search for peer-reviewed published articles using ABM in each topic area.

Infectious Disease	# of ABM published peer-reviewed articles found
Scopus	314
Web of Science	288
Cross-referenced in both databases	20
Obesity	# of ABM published peer-reviewed articles found
Scopus	46
Web of Science	50
Cross-referenced in both databases	13
Tobacco	# of ABM published peer-reviewed articles found
Scopus	20
Web of Science	31
Cross-referenced in both databases	7

Communicable disease: The Scopus search syntax including Boolean operators used was TITLE-ABS-KEY (("Agent-based Model" OR "Agent-based Models" OR "Agent based") AND ("infectious disease" OR epidemic OR pandemic)) AND (LIMIT-TO (SRCTYPE, "j")) AND (LIMIT-TO (LANGUAGE, "English")) AND (LIMIT-TO (DOCTYPE, "ar")). The Web of Science search syntax used was (TS=("Agent-based Model" OR "Agent-based Models" OR "agent based") AND TS = ("infectious disease" OR epidemic OR pandemic) AND LANGUAGE: (English) AND DOCUMENT TYPES: (Article).

Obesity: **The** Scopus search syntax was TITLE-ABS-KEY (("Agent-based Model" OR "Agent-based Models" OR "agent based") AND (obes* OR overweight OR bmi OR "Body Mass")) AND (LIMIT-TO (SRCTYPE, "j")) AND (LIMIT-TO (LANGUAGE, "English")) AND (LIMIT-TO (DOCTYPE, "ar")). The Web of Science syntax was (TS=("Agent-based Model" OR "Agent-based Models" OR "agent based") AND TS = (obes* OR overweight OR bmi OR "Body Mass")) AND LANGUAGE: (English) AND DOCUMENT TYPES: (Article).

Tobacco Control: **The** Scopus syntax used was TITLE-ABS-KEY (("Agent-based Model" OR "Agent-based Models" OR "Agent based") AND (toba* OR smoking OR tobacco)) AND (LIMIT-TO (SRCTYPE, "j")) AND (LIMIT-TO (LANGUAGE, "English")) AND (LIMIT-TO (DOCTYPE, "ar")). And for Web of Science, the search syntax was (TS=("Agent-based Model" OR "Agent-based Models" OR "agent based") AND TS = (toba* OR smoking OR tobacco)) AND LANGUAGE: (English) AND DOCUMENT TYPES: (Article).

search terms used for each topic, so interested readers can replicate our searches in each database and can update the search results to see how ABM usage has increased in each area.

Table 5.1 presents the results for each of the three topic areas: communicable disease (Section A), obesity (Section B), and tobacco control (Section C). In each case, results are shown for Scopus, Web of Science, and cross-referenced articles.

From this full literature search, we select a handful of example models to describe in detail.

5.3   Example Models: Infectious Disease

Among the subfields of public health research, infectious disease epidemiology was the first to see widespread use of mathematical models (including ABMs). Modeling is particularly appealing in this topic space, since it is difficult (infeasible and often unethical) to conduct experiments to understand the way disease spreads through a population or determine the best policy responses to curb an epidemic. Computational models can serve as *policy laboratories*, representing the spread of a disease *in silico*, and experimenting with different policy responses safely within the confines of a computer.

The earliest models of infectious disease were based on systems of ordinary differential equations (Kermack and McKendrick 1927). The most basic version of these models is the *SIR Model* in which the population is divided into three stocks: Susceptible (S), Infected (I), and Recovered (R). In each time period, the size of these stocks increases or decreases in proportion to an infection rate and recovery rate (agents can only move from S → I and I → R). Despite its simplicity, the SIR model generates several key insights into infectious disease epidemiology:

- Every disease has a reproduction number (R_0), defined as the rate of infection divided by the rate of recovery. The extent of an epidemic depends crucially on R_0. Diseases with $R_0 > 1$ produce epidemics, while diseases with $R_0 < 1$ do not.
- As such, the model demonstrates the importance of interventions that generate reductions in R_0. Vaccinating enough individuals to reduce $R_0 < 1$ creates *herd immunity*.

These models are also called *compartment models* because they rely on the simplifying assumption that all individuals can be classified into "compartments" – e.g. susceptible, infected, and recovered. Within each compartment, agents are indistinguishable. Everyone enters and exits each compartment with the same probability.

This assumption, of course, is likely to be violated in many contexts in ways that create interesting complications for the standard SIR model. First, real population density varies dramatically across different geographies, and human social networks are not random (or static). This means that infection rates, and therefore R_0, are likely to vary depending on the context. Second, real humans who are caught in an epidemic adapt their behavior to avoid the disease. Phenomena such as quarantine and flight can complicate the SIR model's predictions and are difficult to represent as systems of differential equations. Agent-based models, however, are ideal for representing both geography and adaptive behavior (see discussion of this point in Chapter 3). The potential advantages of ABM for the study of communicable disease (and the design of containment policies) led the National Institutes of Health (NIH) to fund a large-scale multiyear modeling network entitled MIDAS (Models of Infectious Disease Agent Study https://www. nigms.nih.gov/Research/SpecificAreas/MIDAS/), which developed and applied a large number of ABMs with high scientific and policy impact. Several of these are described below.

Geography

An epidemic that begins in rural West Virginia is likely to progress very differently than one that begins in Hong Kong, due to the differing densities and topographies of human settlement in each of these contexts. In the former case, a disease may be quite virulent but still fail to spread very far. In the latter, even a less-contagious disease could become a global pandemic. Because traditional SIR models do not incorporate geographic information on human settlement patterns and transportation networks, they do not capture this insight. As such, these models cannot provide guidance on policies that are explicitly geographic in nature (e.g. implementation of quarantines, closing airports, or targeted vaccination campaigns).

Burke et al. (2006) present an agent-based model of smallpox contagion and use it to test the effectiveness of various interventions, varying the model's geospatial features. Unlike the SIR model, which represents disease progression with only three "states," the smallpox ABM simulates multiple stages of a smallpox infection, including incubation period (when the host is contagious, but symptoms remain undetected). Rather than assuming random mixing of the population and a constant infection rate, agents are divided into households and interact only with members of their own household, school classmates, workplace coworkers, or (if necessary) hospital workers. Introducing this geospatial variation allowed the researchers to test a variety of intervention strategies, including contact tracing and selective vaccination. Understanding the effects of these particular interventions is an important contribution because mass vaccination is unlikely to be an effective strategy as a response to a sudden smallpox outbreak.

The Burke model produces a number of important and counterintuitive results. First, it reveals that contact tracing alone is unlikely to be effective in the event of a smallpox outbreak. In an area where individuals commute long distances for work, an epidemic might emerge in one town but take off in a completely different town. Nonrandom mixing makes it difficult to predict the geographic progression of an epidemic. Second, the model highlights the importance of vaccinating important nodes within the network. Absent the model, one might plan to distribute vaccine to elderly individuals. But because such individuals are less likely to commute, they are also less likely to spread the disease across city boundaries. Since the elderly are not central to the contact network, these individuals are actually better off if you selectively vaccinate more central individuals (e.g. hospital workers). Furthermore, the model demonstrates the potential effectiveness of combining *multiple* interventions during a disease outbreak: contact tracing plus the reactive vaccination of hospital workers performed better than any single intervention alone.

Epstein et al. (2007) present a large-scale agent-based epidemiological model for influenza. Modeling over 100 of the largest cities in the world and the air traffic connections between them, the model seeks to understand the likely effect of air travel restrictions in the event of a global flu pandemic. Population data are taken from the US Census Bureau, the United Nations Department of Economic and Social Affairs, the Instituto Brasileiro de Geografia e Estatistica, and others. Travel data comes from a previous study on the worldwide air transportation network. The researchers test travel restriction and vaccination policies, and find that travel restrictions can provide a "small, but important delay in the spread of a pandemic," but only if coupled with vaccination. Absent other disease control measures, airport closures can actually worsen outbreaks by delaying intercity travel until a more favorable season for flu transmission.

Germann et al. (2006) conduct a similar study of influenza mitigation strategies, focusing within the United States. This study is also notable for the size of its agent population: 281 million simulated individuals, each assigned demographic and mobility data from the US Census and Department of Transportation. The demographic data is used to calibrate age-specific influenza attack rates (drawn from historical records of past influenza epidemics), and the transportation data is used to determine contact probabilities. Similar to Epstein et al. (2007), this model also finds that travel restrictions typically only delay outbreaks, rather than prevent them entirely. These policies must be coupled with vaccine policy to effectively reduce outbreaks. Fortunately, the model finds that rapid deployment of vaccines, even if poorly matched with circulating strains, significantly improves outcomes. Multiple simultaneous policies are found to produce the best chance of curbing an influenza epidemic.

Lee et al. (2010) simulate school-closure strategies, using the spread of the 2009 H1N1 influenza pandemic to calibrate their model of flu spread. Similar to the Germann model, agents are assigned demography based on the observed geographic distribution of ages in the US Census, and those ages inform the influenza attack rate. Through this exercise, they make several counterintuitive discoveries. First, they find that closures at the entire school system level do not perform better on average than targeted single school closures. Second, school closure can be counterproductive if not maintained for longer than two weeks. In the model, anything less than eight weeks results in students being returned to school in the midst of an epidemic, *worsening* the overall results.

Behavior

Traditional SIR models make another crucial simplification that ABMs are well suited to relax: agents in these models do not adapt their behavior in response to an epidemic. In a Kermack–McKendrick style SIR model, the infection and recovery rates are properties of the disease, not the agents, and remain the same during the height of an epidemic as they are in the early stages of an outbreak. In real-world epidemics, however, people respond to the disease by becoming afraid and potentially fleeing to new areas or hiding themselves away. These behaviors, in turn, affect a disease's infection rate, so understanding how they operate is critical to developing more plausible models of disease spread.

Responding to this need, Epstein et al. (2008) developed a "coupled contagion" model in which agents may be infected by both disease and fear of the disease. It proceeds like a typical agent-based SIR model, except that agents exposed to nearby sick individuals can become "infected with fear," changing their behavior. Fearful agents might hide in place, dampening the epidemic. Or they might flee, spreading the disease to new areas and amplifying the epidemic's R_0. Agents may also be infected with fear by fearful individuals who are not sick, meaning fear can spread faster than the disease itself. As such, the rate at which fear spreads has a substantial effect on the spread of the disease itself. The models that include behavioral responses of this sort are able to shed new light on empirical (and policy-relevant) puzzles such as multiple waves of infection and nonrandom geographic dispersion following transit lines. The model suggests that any effective policy response to infectious disease must consider behavioral responses and be equipped with tools to counteract unnecessary fear.

5.4 Example Models: Obesity

The etiology of obesity is complex. There is a growing recognition that obesity is caused by a multitude of factors, including social influence (Christakis and Fowler 2007), the food environment, and early childhood factors. As the agent-based models of infectious disease demonstrate, this type of modeling is ideal for capturing nonrandom patterns in geography and social interaction. Researchers have, therefore, increasingly turned to ABM to help understand how these factors shape obesity outcomes (Hammond 2009). The potential of ABM for addressing complexity in obesity led to another NIH-funded network known as ENVISION (https://www.nccor.org/projects/envision/), which funded development of both agent-based modeling and other systems-science modeling efforts.

Burke and Heiland (2007) show that an agent-based model incorporating food prices and social influence can reproduce, with great accuracy, the observed change in US weight distributions from the National Health and Nutrition Examination Survey (NHANES) between 1976 and 2000. Agents attempt to maximize a utility function that balances (i) utility from food consumption and (ii) utility from maintaining the same average body weight as one's peers. As the cost of food decreases, agents increase their food consumption, and social influence reinforces that shift, resulting in a heavier equilibrium distribution of body weight by the year 2000.

Hammond and Ornstein (2014) demonstrate that a process of social influence alone can lead to increases in average body weight over time. If agents "follow the average" (FTA), setting their ideal body type equal to the average body weight of agents in their peer group, then a body mass index (BMI) distribution that is initially right skewed will shift upward over time. Their paper demonstrates empirically that school children's ideal body weight is indeed correlated with that of their peers, and then incorporates this insight into an agent-based model. The FTA result is robust to adding complications like influence spreading over social networks and incorporating a metabolic model translating caloric intake into weight change over time. The ABM can also be calibrated to produce observed changes in BMI over time in empirical panel data, suggesting that this mechanism alone could explain observed increases in body weight.

Beheshti et al. (2017) follow a similar strategy, constructing an ABM in which agents consume calories and expend energy, but each of those choices is subject to influence by members of their social network. Their model is calibrated to match observed weight change in the NLSY79 dataset. Then, using this calibrated model, they demonstrate that the strength of obesity interventions depends on which agents are targeted. Interventions that are equally efficacious at the individual-level have much stronger population level effects if they are targeted at agents that are central to the network. They find that an "influence maximization" algorithm, drawn from the viral marketing literature, produces the best results. (Of course, how to identify these agents in the field is an important practical question.)

Auchincloss et al. (2011) explore the role of residential segregation in creating differences across incomes in healthy eating behaviors. In their ABM, agents select food from either healthy or unhealthy food stores on the basis of price and distance. Agents are segregated by income, and healthy food stores are segregated into the wealthy neighborhoods. They demonstrate that, given this setup, interventions aimed at manipulating low-income agents' *preferences* for healthy food did nothing by themselves to reduce disparities. These policies needed to be coupled with reductions in the price of healthy food or reductions in the segregation of stores and/or income groups.

Traditional models of food choice assume that preferences are exogenous; people like certain foods and dislike others. But where do these preferences come from? Hammond et al. (2012) address this question through agent-based modeling, exploring how early childhood exposure can shape food preferences. In their model, agents "learn" which foods they prefer using a temporal difference learning (TDL) algorithm. Neuroscientists have identified this algorithm as a reward learning model that closely mimics the workings of the brain's dopamine system, which sends reinforcing signals in response to novel, pleasurable stimuli. By exposing agents in the model to a sequence of food choices (represented in the model by "palatability scores"), the ABM uncovers an interesting insight. Agents that are exposed early to low-palatable foods are more likely to prefer them later in life than agents that are exposed to the same quantity of low-palatable foods, but during later stages of learning. This "lock-in effect" highlights the importance of early childhood exposure to healthy foods. It also suggests a rationale for why the observed empirical relationship between food environment and healthy eating is puzzlingly weaker than public health researchers would expect: the most important food environment shaping eating habits may be the childhood food environment.

5.5   Example Models: Tobacco Control

Tobacco remains the leading preventable cause of death in the United States and an important driver of health costs and disparities. The tobacco control field has many policy questions that benefit from modeling, and there has been an explosion of interest in policy-oriented computational modeling by the FDA, NIH, and centers for disease control and prevention (CDC). The FDA gained regulatory authority over tobacco products in 2009, with a requirement to fund research to inform their decision-making. Many cities have also begun to act on their own at the local level and serve as policy innovators.

Much of the focus in this field has been on retailer-focused (point of sale) tobacco control efforts that target changes in retail environment with the goal of shifting smoking behaviors. Key challenges include how to design effective retail interventions that will reduce smoking without worsening disparities within and between communities, how to evaluate potential trade-offs between competing strategies (e.g. zoning vs licensing), and how policy "dose" translates into reach and speed.

Agent-based models are especially well suited to addressing these challenges. They offer the ability to capture rich spatial structures and dynamics (which are central to consideration of the inherently spatial retail-oriented policies); they are adept at modeling adaptive behavior over time (such as adaptive responses by consumers and retailers alike in the face of a shifted retail regulatory environment); and they allow potential comparison of many combinations of real-world policy options in ways difficult to undertake with real-world experiments.

Luke et al. (2017) develop a retail policy ABM called "Tobacco Town" to compare point-of-sale policies and evaluate relative magnitude and speed of impact, distributional effects, potential unintended consequences, and coordination with other built environment policies. The model depicts a simulated town complete with homes, workplaces, schools, and tobacco retailers. The Tobacco Town environment is informed by an extensive battery of empirical data on tobacco retailer density, prices, workplace density, schools, and transportation infrastructure. Agents in the model (adults who are already smokers) travel to and from work, smoke cigarettes each day, and travel to a tobacco retailer when they need to purchase more cigarettes. The model computes, for each agent, the excess travel costs incurred on days when they purchase cigarettes at a retailer.

With those computed travel costs as a baseline, the modelers then implemented a variety of proposed tobacco control policies using the simulation. These include license caps, prohibiting tobacco sales near schools, retailer buffers (requiring some minimum distance between tobacco retailers), tobacco-free pharmacies, and combinations of multiple policies. One major advantage of the ABM is the ease with which it evaluates interventions that are fundamentally geographic in nature. Absent a model, it would be quite difficult to estimate how a reduction in retailer density would impact the typical agent's travel costs. Likewise, it is not intuitive whether a school buffer would be more or less effective than a tobacco-free pharmacies policy. By incorporating empirical data on population, retailers, and school density, Tobacco Town can provide a better sense of the likely effects that these policies would have on the availability of tobacco across a variety of settings.

The Tobacco Town model produces a rich set of results, suggesting that the effect of any given policy is likely to depend on the context. In suburban settings, caps on retail licenses were an effective policy for reducing retailer density and increasing travel costs. In dense, urban environments, however, these retailer caps did not produce meaningful cost increases. Even in the most extreme version of that policy (cutting tobacco retailers by 50%), the environment was still sufficiently dense and walkable that tobacco remained easily available. The reverse was true for school buffers: in the dense urban environment, buffers create a tobacco-free lagoon, increasing travel costs for select agents. But in suburban environments, a 1500-ft buffer means little to agents that are primarily commuting by automobile. Given this context conditionality, policies that combined multiple interventions performed the best at reducing tobacco availability, regardless of the town type.

5.6 Conclusions

Although the use of ABM in public health is relatively new, its growth has been impressive. Four IOM reports (IOM (The Institute of Medicine) 2010, 2012, 2013; IOM and NRC (National Research Council) 2015) and five NIH-funded scientific networks[1] have engaged deeply with the use of agent-based models for population

---

1 These include Models of Infectious Disease Agent Study (MIDAS), the National Collaborative on Childhood Obesity Research (NCCOR), the Cancer Intervention and Surveillance Modeling Network (CISNET), the Interagency Modeling and Analysis Group (IMAG), and the Network on Inequality, Complexity, and Health (NICH).

health in the past decade. In addition to the early uses in infectious disease, obesity, and tobacco, recent work has just begun to use ABM to explore other health disparities (Kaplan et al. 2017), including some very preliminary work addressing social determinants of health that are farther from direct behavior and disease outcomes than the bulk of published literature described here. As we argue in the following chapters, we believe that the use of ABM to study social determinants of health is particularly promising and expect this relatively unexplored area of research to grow rapidly in the coming years.

References

Auchincloss, A.H., Riolo, R.L., Brown, D.G. et al. (2011). An agent-based model of income inequalities in diet in the context of residential segregation. *American Journal of Preventive Medicine* 40 (3): 303–311.

Beheshti, R., Jalalpour, M., and Glass, T.A. (2017). Comparing methods of targeting obesity interventions in populations: an agent-based simulation. *SSM-Population Health* 3: 211–218.

Burke, M.A. and Heiland, F. (2007). Social dynamics of obesity. *Economic Inquiry* 45 (3): 571–591.

Burke, D.S., Epstein, J.M., Cummings, D.A. et al. (2006). Individual-based computational modeling of smallpox epidemic control strategies. *Academic Emergency Medicine* 13 (11): 1142–1149.

Christakis, N.A. and Fowler, J.H. (2007). The spread of obesity in a large social network over 32 years. *New England Journal of Medicine* 357 (4): 370–379.

Epstein, J.M., Goedecke, D.M., Yu, F. et al. (2007). Controlling pandemic flu: the value of international air travel restrictions. *PLoS One* 2 (5): e401.

Epstein, J.M., Parker, J., Cummings, D. et al. (2008). Coupled contagion dynamics of fear and disease: mathematical and computational explorations. *PLoS One* 3 (12): e3955.

Germann, T.C., Kadau, K., Longini, I.M. et al. (2006). Mitigation strategies for pandemic influenza in the United States. *Proceedings of the National Academy of Sciences of the United States of America* 103 (15): 5935–5940.

Hammond, R.A. (2009). Complex systems modeling for obesity research. *Preventing Chronic Disease* 6 (3): A97.

Hammond, R.A. and Ornstein, J.T. (2014). A model of social influence on body mass index. *Annals of the New York Academy of Sciences* 1331 (1): 34–42.

Hammond, R.A., Ornstein, J.T., Fellows, L.K. et al. (2012). A model of food reward learning with dynamic reward exposure. *Frontiers in Computational Neuroscience* 6: 82.

IOM (The Institute of Medicine) (2010). *Bridging the Evidence Gap in Obesity Prevention: A Framework to Inform Decision Making* (eds. S.K. Kumanyika, L. Parker and L.J. Sim). Washington, DC: The National Academies Press.

IOM (The Institute of Medicine) (2012). *Accelerating Progress in Obesity Prevention: Solving the Weight of the Nation* (eds. D. Glickman, L. Parker, L.J. Sim, et al.). Washington, DC: The National Academies Press.

IOM (The Institute of Medicine) (2013). *Evaluating Obesity Prevention Efforts: A Plan for Measuring Progress* (eds. L.W. Green, L. Sim and H. Breiner). Washington, DC: The National Academies Press.

IOM and NRC (National Research Council) (2015). *A Framework for Assessing Effects of the Food System* (eds. M.C. Nesheim, M. Oria and P.T. Yih). Washington, DC: The National Academies Press.

Kaplan, G.A., Diez Roux, A.V., Simon, C.P. et al. (eds.) (2017). *Growing Inequality: Bridging Complex Systems, Population Health, and Health Disparities*. Washington, DC: Westphalia Press.

Kermack, W.O. and McKendrick, A.G. (1927). A contribution to the mathematical theory of epidemics. *Proceedings of the Royal Society A* 115 (772): 700–721.

Lee, B.Y., Brown, S.T., Cooley, P. et al. (2010). Simulating school closure strategies to mitigate an influenza epidemic. *Journal of Public Health Management and Practice* 16 (3): 252–261.

Luke, D.A., Hammond, R.A., Combs, T. et al. (2017). Tobacco town: computational modeling of policy options to reduce tobacco retailer density. *American Journal of Public Health* 107 (5): 740–746.

6

Section Summary

Ross A. Hammond

Center on Social Dynamics & Policy, The Brookings Institution, Washington, DC, USA
Brown School, Washington University in St. Louis, St. Louis, MO, USA
The Santa Fe Institute, Santa Fe, NM, USA

This section of the book (Chapters 3–6) has focused on agent-based modeling (ABM), first describing the technique in more detail and then providing numerous concrete examples with a focus on empirically oriented models in fields related to the social determinants of health.

Chapter 3 provided the basic ABM terminology and discussed the technical underpinnings of the technique, along with some history of its use across fields (from biology and social sciences into public health). It introduced the PARTE framework for explicating and comparing ABMs and described an eight-step process that most scientific projects using ABM follow.

Chapter 4 described the scale of ABM use within social science and highlighted three specific case studies of the use of ABM in social science to shed new light on an empirical puzzle. The models that were chosen for more detailed exposition not only highlighted the topic areas of particular interest for social epidemiology but also illustrated three important best practices in ABM design and analysis: the value of simplicity, the value of interdisciplinarity, and the importance of a strong motivating research question. For two of the ABMs described in the chapter, a literature search was conducted to give a sense of the subsequent modeling and empirical work each inspired.

Chapter 5 quantified the growing use of ABM within the public health literature and then highlighted a number of specific examples of empirically oriented ABMs within three domains in which ABM use has been most prevalent: communicable disease, tobacco control, and obesity prevention. The examples also provided illustrative insights into several specific strengths of ABM that may be most relevant for studying social determinants of health – its ability to represent social interactions, spatial structure, and policy contexts.

Although few examples exist to date of ABM applied directly and explicitly to social determinants of health beyond behavioral or disease outcomes, we have argued that this application area has high potential and can leverage the same advantages of the ABM technique laid out in Chapter 3 and illustrated in more detail in Chapters 4 and 5. Here, we conclude the ABM section of the book with an expanded discussion of the use of ABM for policy purposes. We also outline several key gaps that remain in moving ABM work ahead in social epidemiology and the study of the social determinants of health.

6.1   Past Use of ABM for Public Policy Translation

The ABM approach offers a number of potential advantages as a decision aid in a policy setting. First, it permits simulation of situations for which conducting real-world experiments is not feasible (for ethical, cost, or other practical considera-tion). Second, by making explicit many of the assumptions, pathways, and uncertainties involved, models can help decision-makers revisit and discuss implicit mental models that may be driving the decision process. ABM can pro-vide a particularly accessible way to communicate complex dynamics to a group with mixed disciplinary or nontechnical backgrounds. Finally, ABM can help uncover potentially unanticipated (and perhaps unwanted) adaptive system responses that a policy or intervention might trigger and can also uncover distri-butional implications (across individuals, contexts, or time) that any given policy might have.

In general, ABMs that inform policy fall into three distinct categories: prospec-tive policy models, retrospective policy models, and indirect policy models. Prospective policy models (*ex ante* models) help to inform the design of policies or interventions by elucidating their potential effects. These models simulate key dynamic mechanisms in a system and have explicit representations of one or more policy choices; thus, they allow comparison of policy options within the simulated system. In this way, a prospective policy-oriented ABM can identify potential trade-offs or synergies between extant policy choices and can sometimes also help discover previously unnoticed strategies for intervention into a system.

Good examples of prospective policy models from within public health come from the MIDAS work (Burke et al. 2006; Epstein 2004, 2009; Eubank et al. 2004; Ferguson et al. 2006; Germann et al. 2006; Lee et al. 2010; Longini et al. 2005, 2007; Yang et al. 2009) and the Tobacco Town work (Luke et al. 2017), both dis-cussed in Chapter 5. Outside of public health, prospective policy-oriented ABMs have appeared in fields including disaster preparedness (Epstein et al. 2011), retirement policy (Axtell and Epstein 1999), anticorruption interventions (Hammond 2008), agricultural production policies (Berger and Troost 2014), and energy markets (Brady et al. 2012). This type of application for ABM has also appeared in the private sector (e.g. for consideration of changes to logistics, mar-keting, or strategy) (Frederick 2013; North et al. 2010; Rand and Rust 2011).

Retrospective policy-oriented ABMs simulate policies which have already been put into place in the real world to uncover reasons for (retrospectively observed) success or failure. They leverage the ability of ABM to provide insight into complex and dynamic mechanisms that are at work in a system which may not be directly observable, for which data may be missing, or which may be interacting with other mechanisms. ABM can help with causal inference in such circumstances and can also help to understand differential success of a policy or intervention across subpopulations or contexts, which may aid in scaling or translation. Retrospective use of ABM to understand differential success of policies and interventions in public health is relatively rare – one example can be found in Gillman (2014). Examples of this use are more widespread in social science, including work in electoral systems (Laver 2005; Laver and Sergenti 2011) and economics of systemic risk in the housing market (Geanakoplos et al. 2012).

Indirect influence on policy or decision-making may also come from ABMs, even when consideration of policy choices is not an explicit goal. A common use of ABM – understanding etiology driven by bidirectional relationships between system structure and individual behavior over time – can yield discoveries with important implications for policy. These might include identification of key leverage points, mechanisms, or windows of opportunity for intervention. Examples include the obesity etiology work discussed in Chapter 5 (Hammond et al. 2012; Hammond and Ornstein 2014). Social science examples include work on the drivers of segregation discussed in Chapter 4 (Bruch and Mare 2006; Xie and Zhou 2012) and work on the underlying mechanisms that may explain the ubiquity of ethnocentrism (Hammond and Axelrod 2006).

6.2 Bridging Gaps to Advance Agent-Based Modeling of Social Determinants of Health

The use of ABM to better understand the social determinants of health and to improve health outcomes and equity is particularly promising. Some nascent work of this sort is already underway. For ABM to reach its full potential in this space, attention must be paid to addressing gaps in three important areas: (i) data and data usage, (ii) theories of individual behavior, and (iii) training.

Data and Data Usage

Early work in ABM was constrained by the relative paucity of two particular types of data: repeated longitudinal observations of individual-level behavior or decision-making in large heterogeneous populations (to inform P, A, and R for an agent population in ABM as described in the PARTE framework in Chapter 3) and rich contextual data such as ecological momentary assessment (to inform T and E in that framework). In the past decade, there has been an explosion of new forms and sources of data, including many data sources of these exact two types. However, as modelers work to make use of these new data sources, several key questions remain unresolved.

First, there are unavoidable practical trade-offs between maximizing data granularity and managing data magnitude. Given these, what are the best ways for any particular ABM designer to articulate the level of granularity really needed for the model? Are there general guidelines for ABMs in general or in specific topic areas (such as social determinants of health) that the field might be able to articulate to guide data collection?

Second, since collection of contextual information comes with important costs not only for measurement but for managing privacy, what types of context should be prioritized for any particular ABM effort – environmental, social, biological, or other? Again, might the field develop general guidelines for ABMs of particular types? Relatedly, how can data sets that include detailed, longitudinal, and contextual individual level observations be made widely accessible across multiple researchers or models while managing the very difficult privacy concerns they raise?

As the "big data" revolution continues, these and other related questions will become increasingly pressing for data users, including agent-based modelers. Bringing ABM to full fruition in the study of the social determinants of health will almost certainly involve developing clear answers for at least some of these topics.

Theories of Individual Behavior

A second set of important gaps concerns theories of individual behavior and decision-making suitable for incorporation into agent-based models of the social determinants of health. Many of the dominant social science models of decision-making (such as rational choice) are limited in their ability to handle social and environmental influences that coevolve with behavior, while many of the theories of health behavior are not adequately operationalized to implement into a quantitative mechanistic model such as an ABM (Bruch et al. 2014). In addition, a great many of the theoretical constructs across disciplines are focused on the cognitive system and ignore other biological systems that influence behavior and which can be easily incorporated into ABM with sufficient theoretical support (Hall et al. 2014).

Early ABM work in social science and public health often employed either "simple heuristic" rules for agent or standard rational choice formulations from neoclassical economics. Although all models involve simplification as they abstract from the real world, application of ABM to complex behaviors and outcomes that may involve many different inputs, social influence, and noncognitive systems may require more sophisticated representations of individual behavior and decision-making. Active efforts to develop stronger microfoundations for ABM are underway in a number of areas. One promising line of work draws on evidence from marketing science on how humans make decisions in large and multifaceted choice sets (Bruch et al. 2016; Bruch and Feinberg 2017). Another approach involves building into ABM noncognitive models from neuroscience (Epstein 2013; Hammond et al., 2012; Hall et al.,2014). The growing availability of richer individual-level longitudinal data is likely to facilitate development of such models in future.

Training

A third set of challenges surrounds training. There are still few formal resources (books or curricular materials) for training in ABM even within academia,[1] and there are far fewer aimed at other important audiences such as policymakers. This book begins to address this gap in part, but more work is clearly needed to ensure best practices and techniques for the successful use of ABM proliferate. Training is needed not only for practitioners (modelers), but also different training is needed for other researchers who will work in teams with modelers and for end users of models (including policymakers).

References

Axtell, R. and Epstein, J.M. (1999). Coordination in transient social networks: an agent-based computational model on the timing of retirement. In: *Behavioral Dimensions of Retirement Economics* (ed. H. Aaron). Washington, D.C.: Brookings Institution Press.

Berger, T. and Troost, C. (2014). Agent-based modeling of climate adaptation and mitigation options in agriculture. *Journal of Agricultural Economics* 65 (2): 323–348.

Brady, M., Sahrbacher, C., Kellermann, K. et al. (2012). An agent-based approach to modeling impacts of agricultural policy on land use, biodiversity and ecosystem services. *Landscape Ecology* 27 (9): 1363–1381.

Bruch, E.E. and Feinberg, F. (2017). Decision making in social environments. *Annual Review of Sociology* 43: 207–227.

---

1 At the time of the writing of this book, some notable online resources for introductory training to ABM were becoming available. These include https://www.santafe.edu/engage/learn/courses/introduction - agent-based-modeling and https://simulatingcomplexity. wordpress.com/category/tutorials/.

Bruch, E.E. and Mare, R.D. (2006). Neighborhood choice and neighborhood change. *American Journal of Sociology* 112 (3): 667–709.

Bruch, E.E., Hammond, R.A., and Todd, P.M. (2014). Co-evolution of decision-making and social environments. In: *Emerging Trends in the Social and Behavioral Sciences* (eds. R. Scott and S. Kosslyn). Hoboken, NJ: Wiley.

Bruch, E.E., Feinberg, F., and Lee, K.Y. (2016). Extracting multistage screening rules from online dating activity data. *Proceedings of the National Academy of Sciences of the United States of America* 113: 10530–10535.

Burke, D.S., Epstein, J.M., Cummings, D.A. et al. (2006). Individual-based computational modeling of smallpox epidemic control strategies. *Academic Emergency Medicine* 13 (11): 1142–1149.

Epstein, J.M. (2004). *Toward a Containment Strategy for Smallpox Bioterror: An Individual-Based Computational Approach*. Washington, D.C.: Brookings Institution Press.

Epstein, J.M. (2009). Modeling to contain pandemics. *Nature* 460 (7256): 687–687.

Epstein, J.M. (2013). *Agent Zero*. Princeton: Princeton University Press.

Epstein, J.M., Pankajakshan, R., and Hammond, R.A. (2011). Combining computational fluid dynamics and agent-based modeling: a new approach to evacuation planning. *PLoS One* 6 (5): e20139.

Eubank, S., Guclu, H., Kumar, V.A. et al. (2004). Modeling disease outbreaks in realistic urban social networks. *Nature* 429 (6988): 180–184.

Ferguson, N.M., Cummings, D.A., Fraser, C. et al. (2006). Strategies for mitigating an influenza pandemic. *Nature* 442 (7101): 448–452.

Frederick, R. (2013). Agents of influence. *Proceedings of the National Academy of Sciences of the United States of America* 110 (10): 3703–3705.

Geanakoplos, J., Axtell, R., Farmer, J. et al. (2012). Getting at systemic risk via an agent-based model of the housing market. *American Economic Review* 102 (3): 53–58.

Germann, T.C., Kadau, K., Longini, I.M. et al. (2006). Mitigation strategies for pandemic influenza in the United States. *Proceedings of the National Academy of Sciences of the United States of America* 103 (15): 5935–5940.

Gillman, M.W. (2014). Systems science to guide implementation of whole-of-community childhood obesity interventions. Paper presented at The Power of Programming 2014 – Developmental Origins of Adiposity and Long-term Health Conference (13–15 March 2014). Munich, Germany.

Hall, K.D., Hammond, R.A., and Rahmandad, H. (2014). Dynamic interplay among homeostatic, hedonic, and cognitive feedback circuits regulating body weight. *American Journal of Public Health* 104 (7): 1169–1175.

Hammond,R.A. (2008). Endogenous dynamics of corruption. Brookings Institution Center on Social and Economic Dynamics Paper 19.

Hammond, R.A. and Axelrod, R. (2006). The evolution of ethnocentrism. *Journal of Conflict Resolution* 50 (6): 926–936.

Hammond, R.A. and Ornstein, J.T. (2014). A model of social influence on body mass index. *Annals of the New York Academy of Sciences* 1331 (1): 34–42.

Hammond, R.A., Ornstein, J.T., Fellows, L.K. et al. (2012). A model of food reward learning with dynamic reward exposure. *Frontiers in Computational Neuroscience* 6: 82.

Laver, M. (2005). Policy and the dynamics of political competition. *American Political Science Review* 99 (2): 263–281.

Laver, M. and Sergenti, E. (2011). *Party Competition: An Agent-Based Model*. Princeton, NJ: Princeton University Press.

Lee, B.Y., Brown, S.T., Korch, G. et al. (2010). A computer simulation of vaccine prioritization, allocation, and rationing during the 2009 H1N1 influenza pandemic. *Vaccine* 28 (31): 4875–4879.

Longini, I.M. Jr., Halloran, M.E., Nizam, A. et al. (2007). Containing a large bioterrorist smallpox attack: a computer simulation approach. *International Journal of Infectious Diseases* 11 (2): 98–108.

Longini, I.M., Nizam, A., Xu, S. et al. (2005). Containing pandemic influenza at the source. *Science* 309 (5737): 1083–1087.

Luke, D.A., Hammond, R.A., Combs, T. et al. (2017). Tobacco town: computational modeling of policy options to reduce tobacco retailer density. *American Journal of Public Health* 107 (5): 740–746.

North, M.J., Macal, C.M., Aubin, J.S. et al. (2010). Multiscale agent-based consumer market modeling. *Complexity* 15 (5): 37–47.

Rand, W. and Rust, R.T. (2011). Agent-based modeling in marketing: guidelines for rigor. *International Journal of Research in Marketing* 28 (3): 181–193.

Xie, Y. and Zhou, X. (2012). Modeling individual-level heterogeneity in racial residential segregation. *Proceedings of the National Academy of Sciences of the United States of America* 109 (29): 11646–11651.

Yang, Y., Sugimoto, J.D., Halloran, M.E. et al. (2009). The transmissibility and control of pandemic influenza a (H1N1) virus. *Science* 326 (5953): 729–733.

Part III

Microsimulation Modeling

7

Concepts and Methods for Microsimulation Modeling in the Social Sciences

Gerlinde Verbist[1] and Hilde Philips[2]

[1] *Centre for Social Policy, University of Antwerp, Antwerpen, Belgium*
[2] *Centre for General Practice, University of Antwerp, Antwerpen, Belgium*

7.1   Introduction

There are different methods for studying and assessing social and economic policies, at both the micro and macro levels. Microsimulation modeling encompasses a wide range of techniques that operate at the microlevel (i.e. individual decision units) and apply rules to simulate changes in the state of these units or in their behavior. A microsimulation model is a representation of a socioeconomic reality; its purpose is to gain insight into the consequences of proposed policy changes and is therefore a tool for *ex ante* policy analysis. The main advantage of such a model is that it allows one to focus quite accurately on the policy objectives, the tools employed, and the structural changes experienced by those to whom the measures apply. Unlike a macromodel, a microsimulation model allows one to simulate individual decision units. These decision units may be individuals, households, firms, governmental units, etc. Regulations are incorporated into the model as accurately as possible so that the impact on the individual characteristics of a decision unit becomes apparent; the impact of policy rules may, after all, vary considerably for the different units.

Microsimulation modeling in social sciences goes back to the pioneering work of Guy Orcutt (1957) who calls for a new type analytical tool to study the socioeconomic system that "could perform a useful function by increasing the range of predictions that are feasible, by facilitating and improving prediction, by facilitating and improving testing of hypotheses, and by furnishing guidance in selection of research efforts" (1957, p. 121). Before the 1950s, the use by social scientists of the simulation technique was very rare (Orcutt 1960). The amount of research that develops and uses microsimulation modeling has increased considerably

New Horizons in Modeling and Simulation for Social Epidemiology and Public Health, First Edition. Daniel Kim.
© 2021 John Wiley & Sons, Inc. Published 2021 by John Wiley & Sons, Inc.

since the 1980s, thanks to the advent of (large-scale) microlevel databases and powerful computing facilities. Initially, most models were developed and applied among policymakers and academic researchers in the domain of cash transfers and income tax policies. Gradually, this has also extended to other fields, and currently, microsimulation models are used for researching a wide range of public policy domains, such as social policies, taxation, transportation, and health and long-term care.

In this chapter, we discuss the different concepts and methods that are used for microsimulation modeling in social sciences. We start with a discussion of the different methodological choices a microsimulation analyst faces, thereby providing an overview of different types of microsimulation models. Models can be static in nature or can be enriched with different dimensions, such as behavioral reactions, temporal changes, and spatial dimensions. Next, we discuss the different types of input information that is used for these models, distinguishing between constructed and reported data. Finally, we briefly discuss the different domains in which these models are used, thereby illustrating the multi- and interdisciplinary nature of the microsimulation domain.

7.2 Methodological Choices

We can distinguish between different types of microsimulation models by linking them to the methodological choices made. The literature traditionally refers to two types of models, notably static and dynamic models (see Harding 1996; Li et al. 2014a,b); however, this dichotomic distinction does not do justice to the variety of techniques that have been developed and that are used in this domain. In practice, the distinction between the different types has become less relevant (Figari et al. 2015), as modern microsimulation analysis often combines elements of different modeling approaches, depending on the question being addressed. We make a broader typology and discuss the following methodological choices made when developing or using a model and differentiate according to the incorporation of different dimensions:

- Static models;
- Behavioral dimension;
- Time dimension;
- Spatial dimension;
- Macrodimension.

We discuss these different dimensions, starting from the most basic type of model: static models.

Static Models

With static models, the characteristics of the microunits do not change. These models are basically arithmetic, which means that they do not include any changes in behavior or aging. These are models that, in the domain of tax–benefit microsimulations, calculate what disposable income would be for each income unit in the dataset, given the characteristics and the tax–benefit policy rules in place. These models are very suitable to calculate the first-order effects of the existing or alternative policies. Typical questions that can be answered are: What would be the distributive impact of an increase in tax rates? What would the impact be on child poverty if child benefit eligibility were to be expanded? The answer to these questions gives typically "day-after effects" (i.e. without accounting for behavioral or aging effects) on the public budget, inequality and poverty indicators, and work incentives. These models are highly relevant for policymakers and hence are also developed by public administrations. Static models have been used around the globe for a wide range of policy applications (see also Chapter 8).

Incorporating the Behavioral Dimension

Policies do not only have an impact the day after, as static models basically assume, but they also affect human behavior. Behavior of microunits can be affected in various domains, notably labor supply, consumption, housing decisions, financial investment, family formation, mobility, etc. By including such reactions, the scope of the evaluation can be enlarged to include second-order effects. One of the challenges of the previous decades in microsimulation modeling has been to incorporate such microunit behavioral reactions in adequate ways. On the one hand, deciding whether or not to incorporate this dimension depends on the availability of necessary information and data to model such response; on the other hand, the (expected) importance of such reactions is also relevant: if reactions will only be marginal (e.g. because there are restrictions imposed on the ways people can react), then it may be a good decision not to invest in this dimension.

Most of the modeling efforts have concentrated on the topic of labor supply, where over the past decades, major steps have been taken by developing microeconometric models of individual preferences. The start of the use of microsimulation techniques to compute labor supply responses is situated in the early 1980s (see Arrufat and Zabalza 1986; Zabalza 1983). Labor supply reactions have been introduced into microsimulation tax–benefit models since the mid-1990s. Aaberge and Colombino 2014 present a good overview of the different modeling strategies that are (or have been) adopted in modeling labor supply. They focus on "how to develop models that permit a flexible and realistic representation of complicated budget and opportunity sets and allow for a rich representation of households' and opportunities' heterogeneity" (Aaberge and Colombino (2014), p. 170). Examples of modeling labor supply reactions in the framework of tax–benefit policies are provided in Chapter 8.

Incorporating the Time Dimension

The time dimension in microsimulation models is incorporated for several reasons. One reason is to keep the model up to date, typically because input data used are made available with a certain time lag and are hence historical. Thus, by aging the data, the outcomes of the model can be made up to date. Another reason is to evaluate the impact of current measures on future populations, i.e. to provide projections.

There are various ways of incorporating the time dimension. A first way is the process of static aging. *Static aging* involves two different adjustments of the data, notably reweighting and uprating. With reweighting, the weight attached to each unit in the data is changed in order to reflect differences in the composition of the population. If, for example, the share of persons aged 60 or more has increased from 25 to 28% between the time of the data collection and the moment of analysis, this may be incorporated by increasing the weight of persons aged 60 or more. Reweighting is typically used to age sample surveys by a certain number of years in order to bring them up to date or to make projections of the budget in the near future; it has far less been used for projections over a longer time frame, such as 20 years (Harding 1996). Uprating or indexation is needed when there are differences in the period of analysis. This means that monetary amounts are adjusted to changes over time to account for, e.g. income growth or inflation. For indexing income data, two choices can be made (Li et al. 2014a): either income levels are calibrated to aggregate information from National Accounts, or indices are used to account for changes in external control totals (e.g. using consumer prices indices or different indices for different income components if they evolve in a different way in the real world). Static aging techniques can also be used for short- or medium-term projections: using projections of macroaggregates, the distribution of the population can be adjusted to reflect future distributions.

Given that only limited information on demographic and economic trends is considered, static aging is usually not recommended for projections over the longer term but is more appropriate for short-term projections (Dekkers 2012; Dekkers and Liègeois 2012). Immervoll et al. (2005) define static aging techniques as "methods attempting to align the available micro-data with other known information (such as changes in population aggregates, age distributions or unemployment rates), without modeling the processes that drive these changes (e.g. migration, fertility, or economic downturn)."

Dynamic aging, in contrast, models the processes and more specifically those in the population structure; it is a more appropriate tool for longer term projections. A dynamic microsimulation model typically simulates intertemporal transitions in the population, thus modeling the evolution of individual and household characteristics (e.g. age) as well as their behavior and specific life events over time (e.g. birth, marriage, education, and labor market participation). This changing structure can be combined in the model with evolutions in market mechanisms, tax–benefit policies, and the macroeconomic environment. Li et al. (2014b) describe the dynamic models that have been developed, as well as the methodological choices that builders of these models face. In the literature, a distinction is made between cohort models and population models (Harding 1993). Cohort models simulate processes of one cohort over a long time period, while population models simulate the transitions of a cross section of the population over a defined period of time. As Li et al. (2014b) point out, this distinction has become less relevant due to enhanced computational capacity and better data: cohort models were in general used to reduce computing costs, as simulating whole lifetimes for the entire population was very costly. Hence, population models are nowadays considered to be more useful for applied research. The dynamic aging process can take two forms, notably cross-sectional dynamic aging or longitudinal dynamic aging. Cross-sectional dynamic aging occurs when all individuals are updated before moving to the next time period, while longitudinal dynamic aging simulates all time periods for one unit, and this consecutively for all individuals. While cross-sectional aging allows for the matching and interactions between individuals in the dataset, longitudinal aging needs to resort to creating artificial individuals for the sole purpose of forming a partnership, which is an important distinction. Consequently, modelers in general resort to cross-sectional aging if they want to simulate household characteristics in population models (Li et al. 2014b). Methods used to model the different life stages of the relevant microunits within dynamic models include the calculation of transition probabilities and Monte Carlo techniques.

Incorporating the Spatial Dimension

Apart from the time dimension, the spatial dimension is also relevant as social phenomena are geographically heterogeneous. With spatial microsimulation models, one can incorporate the spatial dimension, building further on traditional microsimulation frameworks. This dimension refers to the need for small area demographic and socioeconomic data to support policy planning and research. Small area geographical information can be derived from Census data, but as a Census is, in most countries, usually conducted every 10 years, there is often a data gap for researchers and planners who need such information for intervening years. Filling this gap can be done using spatial microsimulation (Tanton and Clarke 2014). The technique dates back to the mid-1980s, where it was used to support health-care planning (Clarke et al. 1984).

Spatial microsimulation models can produce cross-tabulations for small geographic areas (e.g. poverty for specific groups) and can thus be used by policymakers for planning purposes as well as by researchers to investigate spatial disadvantages (see Tanton 2014 for a review of spatial microsimulation methods). A unit record file is created for each small area, which can potentially be linked to other models to derive small area estimates (Tanton and Clarke 2014). For example in Tanton et al. (2009), small area estimates have been linked with a tax–benefit model, which enables to provide small area estimates of tax–benefit policy changes.

Incorporating the Macrodimension

Linking the microsimulation model with a macro framework is the final dimension we discuss here. The aim is to be able to analyze the impact of changes of macroaggregates (e.g. economic growth) on microunits (e.g. households' disposable income). This link has been developed by integrating microsimulation models within a computable general equilibrium (CGE) model. CGE models typically look at the impact of major policy reforms on aggregate or sectoral price levels and on economic growth or on other macroeconomic aggregates such as national income and national consumption. These models, however, ignore processes at the microlevel and the heterogeneity among microunits. These processes may also impact macroaggregates as not all effects are distributed in the same way over different groups. In sum, CGE models ignore the distributive side, which is typically the key strength of microsimulation models.

7.3 Population Scope

The accuracy of the microsimulation results depends on the quality of the data that underlie the model. Various types of input data are being and have been used for microsimulation models. These input data also determine the population scope of the model. We make a distinction here between data that are collected and data that have been constructed for the purpose of microsimulation.

With collected data, we refer to generally large-scale datasets that come from a survey or from administrative sources. *Administrative data* are data collected by public administrations. They are usually considered to be more accurate, to provide more detail, and also to allow for larger sample sizes, thus leading to more precise estimates and the possibility of providing outcomes for specific groups of the population. A disadvantage of such register data may be that the data are not collected for research purposes and that important information may be missing. For instance, tax administrative files may include only those tax units who have filled their tax declaration; this may imply that units who are exempt from filing a tax declaration (e.g. because their incomes are too low) or who have not returned their tax declaration are missing from the data. For estimating labor supply behavioral reactions, education level is a crucial variable, but this is often not included in administrative data. Moreover, these data may pose additional challenges for international comparative research as administrative definitions and practices can differ across countries. Over the past years, several countries have invested in increasing the quality and scope of administrative datasets. Good practices in this field can be found in the North-European countries, where there are high-quality administrative data available for research (e.g. the Finnish tax–benefit model SISU of Statistics Finland runs on a larger set of register data).

Survey datasets are usually set up to be representative of populations. They are often smaller in scale than administrative records but may be richer in terms of the information they provide for microunits (e.g. bringing together income data with education and health characteristics). Given their smaller scale, survey data may also miss part of the income distribution, as often the bottom or the top incomes are underrepresented. However, survey data may capture information that is not available in register data due to non-take-up of benefits or evasion of taxes (for a discussion on the use of survey and register data in poverty research, see Lohmann 2011). Several microsimulation models run on survey data; the European tax–benefit model EUROMOD runs on the European Union Statistics of Income and Living Conditions (EU-SILC). For both administrative and survey data, it may be necessary to update the dataset through uprating and/or reweighting (described in the previous section) as the data often lag some years behind; this may be especially an issue in times of demographic or economic shocks.

Constructed input data can be divided into two types: hypothetical data or synthetic data. **Hypothetical data** refer to the use of specific types of units on which the policy rules run. A model that runs on hypothetical data is especially useful to focus on the functioning and interactions of specific policies. They show very clearly what the impact is of specific policies on specific microunits. Burlacu et al. (2014) present five drivers for the use of this type of model: (i) illustrative purposes; (ii) validation of the policies in the model; (iii) cross-national comparisons; (iv) replacement of insufficient or lack of data; and (v) communication with the public. A well-known example consists of the hypothetical model families which are used by the OECD in tax–benefit calculations (http://www.oecd.org/els/soc/benefitsandwagestax-benefitcalculator.htm). Recently, the hypothetical household tool (HHoT) was developed within EUROMOD, thus enlarging the simulation possibilities of this model (Hufkens et al. 2016). These tax–benefit hypothetical household simulations help to gain a better understanding of the interactions between different tax–benefit policies and to identify trends in tax and benefit levels. Hence, their primary advantage is an illustrative function. Also, they help to validate complex policy models by disentangling the various policy simulation steps for one specific unit. In addition, they are a convenient tool for cross-country comparisons, provided that assumptions are equivalent across countries. As input data are constructed for the model, this also means that hypothetical data models can be used for a wider scope of policies than models based on collected data. For example, if no information in the collected data is available regarding health status, related policies cannot be simulated; by constructing hypothetical microunits according to health status, this may be remedied. Finally, results from hypothetical data models are often easy to communicate to the public, and models that have been developed with a user interface on the internet can allow the public at large to perform their own simulations. By their very nature, hypothetical household simulations cannot be used for distributional analysis, which is possible with the next type of data.

Synthetic data refers to data that is constructed to consist of individuals and households, in which the characteristics of the individuals in aggregate match the known aggregates from another source. This method has been typically used within the domain of spatial microsimulation modeling: one may start from a created population that has a known age/sex distribution and which is then adjusted to reflect other characteristics, such as the known labor force distribution, occupation, and industry; these characteristics are matched in a sequential way (Tanton 2014). The main method used in this context is iterative proportional fit, which constructs a synthetic dataset for a small area using Census tables and joint probability distributions (Birkin and Clarke 1988, 1989; Tanton and Clarke 2014). One of the advantages of this synthetic reconstruction method is that no micro dataset is required; rather, a synthetic one is created (see Tanton 2014).

7.4 Policy Scope

Microsimulation models are used in a wide range of scientific disciplines and for various sorts of policy questions. The domain is clearly multidisciplinary, but also interdisciplinary, as the increased complexity of modeling has often brought together scholars from different backgrounds. A large part of the existing models are tax–benefit models, which relate to cash transfers and taxes. A prominent example of this type of tax–benefit models is EUROMOD, which is a microsimulation platform that includes tax–benefit policies of all European Union countries (Figari et al. 2015; see also Chapter 8). It also has spin-off models for other countries, at different parts of the world (e.g. Namibia, Russia, Serbia, and South Africa). These tax–benefit models are often static in nature; they differ, however, with respect to the scope of policies they include. Models that encompass all tax–benefit policies are rare, given that data are often lacking to compute, for instance contributory benefits (which typically need information over the entire or part of the individual's career).

The policy scope of microsimulation models has expanded gradually over time. There is a growing body of literature on models that are being used to tackle questions relating to demography, geography, transportation choices, environmental issues, and medicine and public health. A more detailed description of models and applications in these domains can be found in Chapters 8 and 9.

7.5 Building a Microsimulation Model

Once the different methodological choices have been made and the policy scope is defined, a model can be built. The basic building blocks of a (static) microsimulation model are the input data, the set of policy rules, and the output data (see Figure 7.1). Depending on the choice of the dimensions that are incorporated, changes in the population structure and the integration of the spatial and macro dimensions can be part of the model.

Input Data Collection and Preparation

We have already discussed the choice of input data in Section 7.3. Often, these data require a certain amount of preparation before they can be integrated into a microsimulation model. This preparation can refer to data cleaning or the

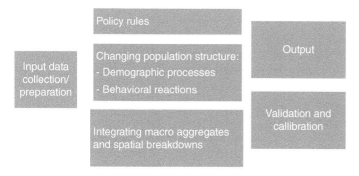

Figure 7.1   Building blocks of a microsimulation model.

imputation of missing data. For tax–benefit models, often a net-to-gross income procedure needs to be included, as many datasets only have net income information, while gross incomes are needed for tax–benefit calculations. Immervoll and O'Donoghue (2001) describe an iterative algorithm to execute this procedure. The updating processes described in Section 7.2 – uprating and reweighting – may also need to be applied, as there is often a lag between the time of data collection and the time of model construction.

Including the Policy Rules

Policy rules are the second major component of microsimulation models in social sciences. Policy rules are a set of computer routines programmed in a generic or a specific computer language, in order to model the relevant legislation. In the case of a tax–benefit model, these refer to a set of parameterized policy rules of the taxes and benefits. This means that the legislation is translated in a sequence of computer routines, which can be adapted to simulate the impacts of alternative tax–benefit policies. As legislation changes over time, the policy rules must be updated regularly, which can be a time- and labor-intensive procedure. Li et al. (2014a) show that an annual update of a tax–benefit model can range from several days to several weeks, depending on the complexity of the tax–benefit system and policy changes.

Changing the Population Structure

If one wants to go beyond first-order effects, it is necessary to provide modules within the model or separate models that account for changes in the population structure. Demographic processes can be integrated through dynamic modeling to provide long-term projections, as discussed in Section 7.2. As Li et al. (2014b) indicate, microsimulation models can incorporate demographic processes using reduced-form statistical models or simple transition matrices. These can be used to simulate process such as family formation, mortality, and fertility. Apart from demographic processes, behavioral reactions could be incorporated to capture the impact of policy structure on human behavior. While different types of behavioral reactions are potentially relevant for a microsimulation model (e.g. consumption, housing and financial investment decisions, and take-up of benefits), most efforts have concentrated on labor supply responses. Such integration of labor supply reactions in microsimulation models requires three components, notably, an arithmetic tax–benefit model to estimate budget constraints, a behavioral model that can be quantified with available or simulated variables, and a mechanism that can predict labor supply under new policy and environmental conditions (Creedy and Duncan 2002; Li et al. 2014b).

Integrating Macroaggregates and Spatial Breakdowns

Depending on the purpose of the model, the macro level and spatial dimensions can be part of its structure. The building of spatial models requires some known aggregates, coming from a Census and/or administrative data, that can be used as a benchmark (Tanton and Clarke 2014). These aggregates, which can relate to demographic, economic, and social variables, form the basis for creating records for each small area. Tanton and Clarke (2014) distinguish between static and dynamic spatial models, and within static models, make a distinction between synthetic reconstruction methods and reweighting approaches, which are distinct ways of simulating the population of a specific area. The inclusion of the macrodimension is in general done by linking microsimulation models with CGE models. As Peichl (2016) and Cockburn et al. (2014) describe, there are two broad ways of linking such models. The first way is to completely integrate the micro and macro models into a joint model. A second approach is to combine the two separate models through interfaces.

Deriving Output Data

In a microsimulation model, the policy rules are applied to the input data, which results in the output dataset. This output dataset contains for every unit the simulated variables, which in the case of tax–benefit modeling are taxes, benefits, and the resulting disposable income. These output data then form the basis to derive relevant indicators, such as inequality and poverty, or work incentives in the cases of tax–benefit models.

Validation and Calibration

On the basis of the output, the model needs to be validated. This can be done by comparing the outcomes with other sources. In the case of a tax–benefit model, this typically entails a comparison of simulated tax and benefit budgets with those of public administrative data. There are, however, many reasons why such a comparison might be hampered. This may be due to characteristics of the available information of the public administrations; for instance, it might be difficult to match the exact categories of taxes and benefits that have been simulated. In addition, some issues relating to the microsimulation modeling itself such as benefit non-take-up and tax evasion may lead to differences in outcomes.

Another aspect that is difficult to incorporate into a microsimulation model is administrative feasibility. Factors relating to administrative feasibility have consequences in terms of the relation between the potential beneficiary and the administration, and therefore also on the process of allocation and take-up of benefits.

7.6 Applications for Policy Making: Illustrations in the Domain of Health

In this section, we illustrate how microsimulation models have been used in the domain of health. We currently live in an era of high-quality health care, with high costs, increasing demand, and decreasing workforce. Policymakers are largely challenged to deal with these evolutions, as they try to keep the balance between qualitative and affordable care. Sustainability must also be considered concerning the decreasing manpower in health care, that is a reality in most countries. Therefore, policymakers now consider a triple aim in health care. The triple aim (Berwick et al. 2008) concept focuses on (i) improving the experience of care (including quality and satisfaction); (ii) improving the health of populations; and (iii) reducing the capita cost of health care. The topics we find in the triple aim policy are exactly the subjects that could benefit from methodologies such as microsimulation models.

As mentioned by Schofield et al. (2014), health is a relatively new application of microsimulation. Nevertheless, health-care services and health policy might be very well served with microsimulation models as they might help to improve the medical profession and the quality of care. This is not only so for policymakers and organization of health-care services (does the health workforce match the need for health care?) but for quality of care and use of guidelines by physicians and other care givers as well. We first provide an overview of selected existing models, and then discuss two different applications.

Microsimulation Models in the Domain of Health

The development and application of microsimulation to health and health policy have expanded considerably over the past decades. Microsimulation models related to health are on the one hand tax–benefit models or broad models of demographic, economic, and welfare processes that include a health module, and on the other hand, purpose-built models with the primary aim of simulating health processes and/or health policies (Lymer et al. 2009; Schofield et al. 2014). Table 7.1 provides an overview of purpose-built health-related models. This table does not give an exhaustive overview of health-related models but illustrates what these models can be used for and which dimensions they incorporate.

For many countries, there now exist microsimulation models related to health issues, but most of them can be found in Australia, which played a pioneering role for these types of models. Most models listed in Table 7.1 are based on survey data. Gathering good-quality data regarding health for microsimulation purposes is complicated. Barriers to date can be found in the huge requirements that are

Table 7.1 Selection of microsimulation health-related models.

Model name	Aims/objectives	Dimensions	Data
HealthandWealth MOD (Australia) Schofield et al. (2011)	Estimate economic impacts of chronic conditions on older workers, aged 45–65 years	Static	Survey of Disability, Ageing and Carers
MedDemandMOD (Australia) Schofield et al. (2012)	Estimate extent of unmet demand for general practitioner services in disadvantaged areas	Static	Australia National Health Survey (NHS)
HEALTHMOD (Australia) Lymer et al. (2011)	Model doctor and medical services	Static aging	Synthetic, derived from Household Expenditure Survey (HES) and National health Survey (NHS)
HealthAgeingMod (Australia) Walker and Calogiuri (2011)	Model links between health risk factors and chronic diseases, taking account of comorbidities	Static aging; health state transitions	National health Survey (NHS), 2003 Survey of Disability Ageing and Carers (SDAC), AusDiab survey
POHEM (Canada) Will et al. (2001)	Compare competing health intervention alternatives	Dynamic	Synthetic, derived from Canadian Community Health Service (CCHS) survey; Additional variables imputed using a range of administrative datasets
COMPARE (USA) Cordova et al. (2013)	Model impact of various policy options on public health insurance coverage	Dynamic, behavioral	Synthetic, derived from Survey of Income and Program Participation (SIPP); Medical Expenditure Panel Survey (MEPS); Kaiser Family Foundation/Health Research and Educational Trust Employer Survey (Kaiser/HRET); Survey of U.S. Businesses (SUSB) and Group Medical Insurance Large Claims Data Base
MoSeS (UK) Birkin et al. (2009)	Model produces microlevel estimates of synthetic individuals including changes in six demographic processes	Dynamic, spatial	British Household Panel Survey; UK census; ONS Mid-Year Estimation and subnational projections; Special Migration Statistics; Vital Statistics
CareMod (Australia) Lymer et al. (2009)	Model regional need for aged care services	Spatial	Survey of Disability, Ageing and Carers, Census small area data
SimSALUD (Austria) Tomintz and Garcia-Barrios (2016)	Model health-related issues for small areas	Spatial	Austrian Health Survey; Census

Source: Schofield et al. (2014) and indicated references.

necessary to access data registers and to gather medical data for other purposes than strictly allowed for caregiving only. Medical data, when linked to personal data, are very sensitive material. Privacy laws, until now, differ between countries, making the use of large-scale databases in different countries very difficult.

Several models have taken a static approach (e.g. HealthandWealthMOD and MedDemandMOD in Australia), while others have included the time dimension. HEALTHMOD and HealthAgeingMod (also for Australia) have applied static aging techniques, while the North-American models POHEM and COMPrehensive Assessment of Reform Efforts (COMPARE) belong to the family of dynamic models. The spatial dimension has been the explicit focus of models such as MoSeS (UK), SimSALUD (Austria), and CareMod (Australia). This illustrates clearly the wide variety in modeling and the attention paid to the different dimensions as described in Section 7.2.

Examples of Applications

Microsimulation models that have been developed have been used for several applications in domains including health expenditure, spatial analysis, mortality, and the health workforce (Schofield et al. 2014; see Chapter 9 for a comprehensive review). Below, we present two examples of applications with health-related microsimulation models, one for the United States (COMPARE) and one for Australia (MedDemandMOD).

One of the recent applications of microsimulation models in the United States is an initiative set up by the RAND Corporation in 2005 to model anticipated health-care policy changes in the United States (Cordova et al. 2013). This resulted in the COMPARE microsimulation model, which has been used to estimate the impact of major policy changes in health care. A prime example of such a policy change is the Affordable Care Act (ACA), which is the US health-care reform that came into effect in 2010. COMPARE is a model in which individuals, firms, and subfamily units (individuals covered by private insurance family plans) consisting of an adult, his or her spouse, and dependent children are considered as the agents. Different characteristics are defined in three categories: endogenous (determined by interactions among the units), exogenous (do not change over the course of the simulation), and variable characteristics (which are allowed to vary during the simulation). COMPARE creates a synthetic representation using three data sources with nationally representative data of individuals, households, and employers and extra data from surveys (see Table 7.1 for an overview of the surveys). The model runs different steps: calibration, simulation of postreform state of the world, and finally the resulting postreform state of the world. This final result is the new equilibrium that originates after the reform. COMPARE enables the model to estimate the impact at both the national and the state levels.

COMPARE has been used to simulate the potential impact of the ACA on overall uninsured rates, enrolment in public programs (e.g. Medicaid), the budgetary cost for the government, etc. (Cordova et al. 2013). The main outcomes of interest are the changes that will take place in the proportion of nonelderly Americans who have insurance coverage, the number of employers that offer health insurance, premium prices, total employer spending, and total government spending. Among nonelderly Americans, the model projected that employer-sponsored insurance coverage would not change after implementation of the ACA. On the contrary, the population on Medicaid and Children's Health Insurance Program (CHIP) and on Individual Exchanges increased with, respectively, 16 and 26 million people (the latter was nonexistent before the ACA). The populations with nongroup and other health insurance coverage and the uninsured decreased with 12 and 29 million people. COMPARE can be used to estimate these effects on each one of the 50 US states.

A second example is the Australian MedDemandMOD, which has been used to study different applications of health care based on socioeconomic inequalities in health. For example, MedDemandMOD uses data from the 2005 National Health Survey of the Australian Bureau of Statistics (Schofield et al. 2012) to investigate the demand for General Practitioner (GP) services in a system with equal utilization of health services relative to need. The authors have used the following determinants for unmet demand: sex, age, regional factors (remoteness), socioeconomic factors (personal income and employment status), and indicators of need (health status) to build the model. They concluded that nationwide, there would be an additional 5% GP visits if the population living in regional areas would have the same access to GP services that those in major cities do. The changes were mainly seen among Australians who are unemployed (19% increase) and people in the lowest personal income tercile (5% increase) and the second tercile (7% increase). The use of GP services by people living in regional areas would become higher than for persons living in major cities; this is a reflection of both the current lack of services and poorer health of rural Australians.

7.7 Conclusions

In this chapter, we have presented how microsimulation modeling can and has been used as a research instrument in the social sciences. Depending on the research question and needs, different types of models have been developed ranging from static first-order models to models that incorporate dimensions of time, behavior, space, and the macroenvironment. We have also briefly discussed some examples of how these models have been applied to health-related issues. Further empirical applications are presented in the next chapter.

References

Aaberge, R. and Colombino, U. (2014). Microsimulation and Labor Supply Models: a survey and an interpretation. In: *Handbook of Microsimulation Modeling*, Contributions to Economic Analysis, vol. 293 (ed. C. O'Donogue), 167–221. Emerald Group Publishing Limited.

Arrufat, J. and Zabalza, A. (1986). Female labor supply with taxation, random preferences, and optimization errors. *Econometrica Econometric Society* 54 (1): 47–63.

Berwick, D., Nolan, T., and Whittington, J. (2008). The triple aim: care, health, and cost. *Health Affairs* 27 (3): 759–769.

Birkin, M. and Clarke, M. (1988). SYNTHESIS – a synthetic spatial information system for urban and regional analysis: methods and examples. *Environment and Planning* 20 (12): 1645–1671.

Birkin, M. and Clarke, M. (1989). The generation of individual and household incomes at the small area level using synthesis. *Regional Studies* 23 (6): 535–548.

Birkin, M., Turner, A., Wu, B. et al. (2009). MoSeS: a grid-enabled spatial decision support system. *Social Science Computer Review* 27 (4): 493–508.

Burlacu, I., O'Donoghue, C., and Sologon, D. (2014). Hypothetical models. In: *Handbook of Microsimulation Modeling* (ed. C. O'Donoghue), 23–46. Emerald Group Publishing.

Clarke, M., Forte, P., Spowage, M., and Wilson, A.G. (1984). A strategic planning simulation model of a district health service system: the in-patient component and results. In: *Third International Conference on System Science in Health Care*, 949–954. Berlin Heidelberg: Springer.

Cockburn, J., Savard, L., and Tiberti, L. (2014). Macro-micro models. In: *Handbook of Microsimulation Modeling* (ed. C. O'Donoghue), 275–304. Emerald Group Publishing.

Cordova, A., Girosi, F., Nowak, S. et al. (2013). The COMPARE microsimulation model and the U.S. affordable care act. *International Journal of Microsimulation* 6 (3): 78–117.

Creedy, J. and Duncan, A. (2002). Behavioural microsimulation with labor supply responses. *Journal of Economic Surveys* 16 (1): 1–39.

Dekkers, G. (2012), The simulation properties of microsimulation models with static and dynamic ageing. A guide into choosing one type of model over the other. Mimeo.

Dekkers, G. and Liègeois, P. (2012), The (dis)advantages of dynamic and static microsimulation. Mimeo.

Figari, F., Paulus, A., and Sutherland, H. (2015). Microsimulation and policy analysis. In: *Handbook of Income Distribution*, vol. 2 (eds. A.B. Atkinson and F. Bourguignon). Amsterdam: Elsevier.

Harding, A. (1993). *Lifetime Income Distribution and Redistribution. Application of a Microsimulation Model*, Contributions to Economic Analysis, vol. 221. Amsterdam: North-Holland.

Harding, A. (ed.) (1996). *Microsimulation and Public Policy*, Contributions to Economic Analysis, vol. 232. Amsterdam: Elsevier North-Holland.

Hufkens T., Leventi C., Rastrigina O., Manios K., Van Mechelen N., Verbist G., Sutherland H. and Goedemé T. (2016). Deliverable 22.2: HHoT: a new flexible Hypothetical Household Tool for tax-benefit simulations in EUROMOD, Leuven, FP7 InGRID project.

Immervoll, H. and O'Donoghue, C. (2001). Imputation of gross amounts from net incomes in household surveys. An application using EUROMOD. EUROMOD Working Paper EM1/01: Essex.

Immervoll, H., Lindstrom, K., Mustonen, E., and Viitamaki, H. (2005). Static data 'ageing' techniques: accounting for population changes in tax-benefit microsimulation models, EUROMOD Working Papers EM7/05, EUROMOD at the Institute for Social and Economic Research.

Li, J., O'Donoghue, C., Loughrey, J., and Harding, A. (2014a). Static models. In: *Handbook of Microsimulation* (ed. C. O'Donoghue), 47–66. Bingley: Emerald.

Li, J., O'Donoghue, C., and Dekkers, G. (2014b). Dynamic models. In: *Handbook of Microsimulation* (ed. C. O'Donoghue), 305–333. Bingley: Emerald.

Lohmann, H. (2011). Comparability of EU-SILC survey and register data: the relationship among employment, earnings and poverty. *Journal of European Social Policy* 21 (1): 37–54.

Lymer, S., Brown, L., Harding, A., and Yap, M. (2009). Predicting the need for aged care services at the small area level: the CAREMOD spatial microsimulation model. *International Journal of Microsimulation* 2 (2): 27–42.

Lymer, S., Brown, L., Harding, A., and Payne, A. (2011). Challenges and solutions in constructing a microsimulation model of the use and costs of medical services in Australia. *International Journal of Microsimulation* 4 (3): 17–31.

Orcutt, G.H. (1957). A new type of socioeconomic system. *Review of Economics and Statistics* 39 (2): 116–123.

Orcutt, G.H. (1960). Simulation of economic systems. *American Economic Review* 50 (5): 893–907.

Peichl, A. (2016). Linking microsimulation and CGE. *International Journal of Microsimulation* 9 (1): 167–174.

Schofield, D., Shrestha, R., Percival, R. et al. (2011). Modeling the cost of ill health in HealthandWealthMOD (Version II): lost labor force participation, income and taxation, and the impact of disease prevention. *International Journal of Microsimulation* 4 (3): 33–37.

Schofield, D.J., Shrestha, R.N., and Callander, E.J. (2012). Access to general practitioner services amongst underserved Australians: a microsimulation study. *Human Resources Health* 10 (1): 1–6.

Schofield, D., Carter, A., and Edwards, K. (2014). Health models. In: *Handbook of Microsimulation Modeling* (ed. C. O'Donoghue), 421–447. Bingley: Emerald.

Tanton, R. (2014). A review of spatial microsimulation methods. *International Journal of Microsimulation* 7 (1): 4–25.

Tanton, R. and Clarke, G.P. (2014). Spatial models. In: *Handbook of Microsimulation Modeling* (ed. C. O'Donoghue), 367–383. Bingley: Emerald.

Tanton, R., Vidyattama, Y., McNamara, J. et al. (2009). Old, single and poor: using microsimulation and microdata to analyse poverty and the impact of policy change among older Australians. *Economic Papers: A Journal of Applied Economics and Policy* 28 (2): 102–120.

Tomintz, M. and Garcia-Barrios, V. (2016). simSALUD – Towards a health decision support system for regional planning. In: *Applied Spatial Modeling and Planning: 392* (eds. J. Lombard, E. Stern and G.P. Clarke). London: Routledge.

Walker, A. and Calogiuri, S. (2011). Cost-benefit model system of chronic diseases in Australia to assess and rank prevention and treatment options. *International Journal of Microsimulation* 4 (3): 57–70.

Will, B., Berthelot, J.-M., Nobrega, K. et al. (2001). Canada's Population Health Model (POHEM): a tool for performing economic evaluations of cancer control interventions. *European Journal of Cancer* 37: 1797–1804.

Zabalza, A. (1983). The CES utility function, non-linear budget constraints and labor supply: results on female participation and hours. *Economic Journal, Royal Economic Society* 93 (37): 312–330.

8

Empirical Evidence Using Microsimulation Models in the Social Sciences

Francesco Figari and Emanuela Lezzi

Department of Economics, University of Insubria, Varese, Italy

8.1 Introduction

This chapter focuses on some empirical evidence in areas of social sciences where microsimulation plays a relevant role both for academic and policy achievements. Building on the concepts and methods defined in Chapter 7, this chapter reviews some important and recent approaches and applications in economics, demography, geography, transport and environmental sciences, and identifies the intersections between the analyses performed in the different areas both in terms of methodology and content.

Furthermore, this chapter highlights the potential overlaps between microsimulation models (as defined in Chapter 7) and agent-based modeling (as defined in the first part of the book), despite the lack of consensus in the literature on a unique definition of the terms "microsimulation" and "agent-based" models across disciplines. In general, microsimulation can be considered an agent-based model if a common notion of agent-based "as atomistic agents whose interactions and reactions within a shared environment determine the overall behaviour of the system" (Mason 2014) is adopted. This is particularly relevant in the context of microsimulation models applied to demographic and transport-related issues. The link between microsimulation and agent-based models is stronger when agent-based computational models "presuppose (realistic) rule of behaviour and try to challenge the validity of the rules by showing whether they can or cannot explain macroscopic regularities" (Billari et al. 2003).

Overall, the academic literature on microsimulation and the applications based on microsimulation models have expanded enormously in the last 20 years along with the spread and development of the methodology. An attempt to cover all relevant publications would be a daunting task and, therefore, we can only refer to the most recent "survey of surveys" as reported in Figari et al. (2015). However

New Horizons in Modeling and Simulation for Social Epidemiology and Public Health, First Edition. Daniel Kim.

a quantitative review of the entries in different literature databases provides a first indication of the relative use of microsimulation models in each field. Any quantification of the research outputs based on a microsimulation model needs to be interpreted very carefully as the identified outputs may likely represent a lower bound of the total number of products and their classification in the different research areas can be, in some cases, quite arbitrary.

Table 8.1 reports the number of entries related to the term "microsimulation" in some of the most used databases in the Social Sciences. Notwithstanding the caveats mentioned above, it is clear that the use of microsimulation techniques is widely applied in particular in transport-related research and in the analysis of tax–benefit policies. The major differences between the number of entries in Web of Science, Scopus and Google Scholar are due to the fact that the latter includes

Table 8.1   Number of entries related to "microsimulation" in social sciences.

Database	2015	2014	2013	2012	2011	2010
Web of science						
Tax–benefit	19	34	33	32	23	24
Demography	4	6	13	10	9	7
Geography	5	6	15	15	20	8
Transport	61	71	90	92	75	46
Environment	1	1	4	2	6	0
Scopus						
Tax–benefit	19	28	26	27	31	29
Demography	13	8	10	6	2	4
Geography	14	9	9	11	7	7
Transport	38	51	45	44	50	38
Environment	1	1	1	2	3	1
Google scholar						
Tax–benefit	1010	994	1070	1090	1000	916
Demography	331	287	326	319	257	256
Geography	1380	1390	1410	1300	1140	1080
Transport	1770	1810	1900	1660	1500	1440
Environment	1970	1990	1960	1840	1660	1510

Notes: Latest access to the databases on 25 March 2016. Entries with the word "microsimulation" or "micro-simulation" either in Title, Abstract or Keywords. In Web of Science and Scopus the numbers refer to unique entries classified by research areas, while in Google Scholar the same entry can be repeated in more research areas.

research products that – although they are publicly available in the form of working/discussion papers, research notes or project reports – do not necessarily end up in indexed publications. Such products, whose quality is not always ensured by a peer review process, are nonetheless an important channel of dissemination of microsimulation research outputs with potential relevant implications for the policy making process.

There are also obvious overlaps among research areas not directly captured by the entries in the table below: most of transport-related research overlaps with geography, spatial, and environmental-related analysis; the analysis of tax–benefit policies related to the ageing population, retirement and caring decisions overlaps clearly with demographic issues. For example, a budgetary and redistributive analysis of a potential or actual reform of the pension system, which is a clear application of microsimulation techniques in the area of tax–benefit policies, might draw on the population projections produced by a demographic microsimulation model or defined internally, taking into account the evolution of the population over time (Borella and Coda Moscarola 2010). Furthermore, in the area of transport analysis, there are clear connections with the simulation of taxes on emissions and their environmental impact (Cingano and Faiella 2013).

Given the number of microsimulation models currently in use and their quick proliferation across the world, any attempt of completing a comprehensive review would be not only daunting, but quickly out-of-date. The interested reader should refer to the existing surveys of models (see Figari et al. (2015) for an overview) and follow the developments of the microsimulation community through the activities of the International Microsimulation Association (IMA) that was established in 2005, and the *International Journal of Microsimulation*, a refereed online journal. However, most of the models are not accessible to external researchers and their use is limited to the ones who built the models. Two exceptions are represented by EUROMOD and TAXSIM.[1]

EUROMOD is the EU-wide tax–benefit microsimulation covering 28 European countries within the same framework, ensuring the consistency and comparability of results. EUROMOD simulates individual and household tax liabilities and

---

1 Other (selected) examples of models, with detailed information available on the respective web pages, used for policy purposes are the following: APPSIM (Australian Population and Policy Simulation Model - http://www.natsem.canberra.edu.au/models/appsim/); STINMOD (Static Incomes Model – Australia - http://www.natsem.canberra.edu.au/models/stinmod/); TAXBEN (The IFS microsimulation tax and benefit model – UK - https://www.ifs.org.uk/publications/572) FEM (Future Elderly model – USA - http://www.rand.org/labor/roybalhp/projects/health_status/fem.html); LIFEPATHS (Canada - http://www.statcan.gc.ca/microsimulation/lifepaths/lifepaths - eng.htm); MIDAS (Microsimulation for the Development of Adequacy and Sustainability – Belgium, Germany, Italy - http://www.plan.be/publications/Publication_det.php?lang=en & TM=30&KeyPub=781).

cash benefit entitlements according to the policy rules in place in each member state from 2005 up to the current year. The interested user can download the model and the underlying data subject to the permission released by the data providers. Baseline systems in EUROMOD have been validated and tested at a micro level (i.e. case-by-case validation) and macro level. For each system simulated in EUROMOD, Country Reports are available on the EUROMOD web pages with background information on the tax–benefit system(s), a detailed description of all tax–benefit components simulated, a general overview of the input data and an extended summary of the validation process. For more information about EUROMOD, see the official website (https://www.iser.essex.ac.uk/euromod) and Sutherland and Figari (2013). In recent years, the EUROMOD framework and language have been used to build microsimulation models for the Balkan countries (i.e. Macedonia and Serbia), South Africa, and Namibia.

TAXSIM is the NBER microsimulation model that calculates US federal and state income taxes (http://www.nber.org/taxsim/). It covers the federal tax system from 1960 and the state systems from 1977 up to the current year. Model calculations are done in the TAXSIM server on the basis of survey data provided by the users in the required format containing different sources of income, deductions and personal characteristics used to calculate tax liabilities. Recent applications are based on the March Current Population Survey, the Survey of Consumer Finance, the Consumer Expenditure Survey and the Panel Study of Income Dynamics, and a library of scripts by previous users is made available for deriving input data from different sources. See Feenberg and Coutts (1993) for more information.

The remainder of the chapter is organized as follows: The first section covers some of the most relevant uses of microsimulation techniques in economics, focusing on the social impact of tax and benefit policies and the use of microsimulation to estimate individual behavior; the second section offers an overview of the use of microsimulation in different social sciences such as demography, geography, transport research, and environmental sciences.

8.2 Microsimulation and Economics

Microsimulation models currently represent one of the most fruitful interactions between economic research and policy-making processes. There is a growing body of microsimulation-informed economic analysis derived from academic research put forward within governments and by other participants in the policy-making process. Within academia, microsimulation is also widely used in applied public economics and quantitative social policy (Figari et al. 2015). First, microsimulation models are a unique tool for conducting ex ante analysis through the simulation of the counterfactual scenarios reflecting alternative policy regimes (Blundell 2012). Second, microsimulation models provide essential inputs for the analysis of the optimal tax design of policies (Blundell and Shepard 2012). Third, microsimulation outputs are used to feed macro-economic models to measure the effects of macro-economic shocks and policies on the well-being of individuals and their families (Bourguignon and Bussolo 2013).

The current state of interaction between economic research and microsimulation is the result of a long relationship which grew with the developments in economic theory, econometric techniques and information technology availability.

As stated by Aaberge and Colombino (2014), such a relationship started as a *conflictual marriage*. Although in principle, Orcutt's proposal would have represented an ideal match between policy relevant modeling and microeconomics, microeconomic theory principles were not considered in Orcutt's project where behavioral relationships were represented through reduced form specifications.

One can identify a period of *divorce* in the 1970s between economics and microsimulation when most of the efforts had been concentrated in the development of static microsimulation models due to the smaller availability of micro data and computer power. Behavioral reactions were left outside the research programmes, but many developments related to microeconomic theory, micro econometric techniques, and policy related awareness pointed to a clear preparation for a re-encounter between microsimulation and economics.

The *re-marriage* has been clearly a successful one since the beginning of the third millennium with a clearer vision of the respective roles of nonbehavioral and behavioral models, of their possible integration and of new methods to extend the nonbehavioral models.

The Social Impact of Tax and Benefit Policies

The first and immediate use of a microsimulation model in the analysis of tax and benefit policies involves calculating the effects of a given policy on household income, considering the consequences for the public budget and analyzing the new budget constraints faced by the individuals that reveal the financial incentives related to different dimensions. Under the new policy, some people might wish to change their behavior with respect to labor supply, saving, fertility and other aspects of individual behavior. Bourguignon and Spadaro (2006) point out the importance of being clear about when these second order effects can and cannot be neglected. In the first case, a "morning after" analysis – as the pure arithmetic effect is often called – is of value in its own right as the first round effect of a given policy is relevant for both individuals and governments.

The great advantage of microsimulation techniques is that they permit analysis of the impact of policy changes on the overall distribution of target variables rather than on specific moments, for example the mean, as it happens using regression techniques or macro models.

First Round Effects on Income Distribution, Public Budget, and Work Incentives

Tax–benefit models provide information on the distribution of household disposable income and its components under various policy scenarios, which allow policy effects to be inferred. These inferences can be made from doing comparisons of different scenarios when the interactions between policies and characteristics of individuals and their families are taken into account. In a series of papers looking at the overall tax–benefit system, Bargain develops and extends a methodology to quantify the relative effect of tax–benefit policy changes over time, by decomposing the overall effect in the contribution of the changes in the tax–benefit structure, in the underlying population and in the distribution of market income (Bargain 2012a, b; Bargain and Callan 2010).

Although the increasing availability of both net and gross incomes collected or imputed in household surveys allows researchers to conduct analysis on the redistributive effects of tax–benefit policies, microsimulation models can show their strength in producing tailored micro-level information on the redistributive aspects of specific tax–benefit policies. Microsimulation methods can often add to the scope and detail of the analysis, focusing on aspects particularly relevant for shaping the income distribution such as the progressivity of the tax system (Verbist and Figari 2014), the replacement incomes and their interactions with taxes and social contributions in Europe (Verbist 2007), certain federal tax provisions and transfer programs in the Unites States (Hungerford 2010), and the incidence of indirect taxes across the distribution of income or expenditures (Decoster et al. 2010).

The financing and budgetary consequences of any policy change are also explored by means of microsimulation models as they enable establishment of relations between economic agents and macro aggregates. In particular, microsimulation models are able to reproduce the heterogeneity in household budget constraints due to the interactions between personal and family characteristics and tax–benefit rules. For example, if the net cost were met by a percentage point increase in all rates of income tax, this increase might also have knock-on effects (e.g. if the assessment of any means-tested benefits depended on after-tax income) and then iterations of the model would be needed to find a revenue-neutral solution to the tax rate increase. The "revenue neutral" package could then be evaluated relative to the pre-reform situation, in terms of its effect on the income distribution and an analysis of gainers and losers.

Any policy change might or might not involve a change in the incentives that individuals face due to their specific budget constraints. Focusing on one of the most obvious areas of analysis, microsimulation models are able to provide a range of indicators of work incentives for the intensive (i.e. work effort) and the extensive labor supply margin (i.e. decision to work), respectively. Marginal effective tax rates (METRs) reflect financial incentives for a working person to increase his work contribution marginally either through longer hours or higher productivity (increasing the hourly wage rate). METRs show the proportion of additional earnings which is taxed away, taking into account not only personal income tax but also social contributions as well as interactions with benefits, e.g. withdrawal of means-tested benefits as private income increases. As reported in Figure 8.1, Jara and Tumino (2013) show the extent to which average METRs and their distributions vary across the European Union.

Participation tax rates (PTR) are conceptually very similar to effective marginal tax rates, indicating the effective tax rate on the extensive margin, i.e. the proportion of earnings paid as taxes and lost due to benefit withdrawal if a person moves from inactivity or unemployment to work. Replacement rates (RR) complement PTRs, showing the level of out-of-work income relative to in-work disposable income (for an example, see Immervoll and O'Donoghue 2004).

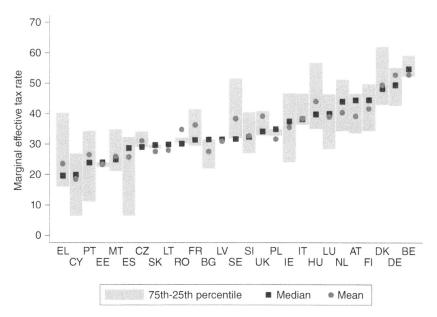

Figure 8.1 Marginal effective tax rates (%) across the European Union, 2007. *Notes:* Official country acronyms: Belgium (BE), Bulgaria (BG), Czech Republic (CZ), Denmark (DK), Germany (DE), Estonia (EE), Ireland (IE), Greece (EL), Spain (ES), France (FR), Italy (IT), Cyprus (CY), Latvia (LV), Lithuania (LT), Luxembourg (LU), Hungary (HU), Malta (MT), Netherlands (NL), Austria (AT), Poland (PL), Portugal (PT), Romania (RO), Slovenia (SI), Slovakia (SK), Finland (FI), Sweden (SE), United Kingdom (UK). *Source:* Jara and Tumino (2013) using EUROMOD.

Redistributive Effects of Tax–Benefit Policies   Figari et al. (2011a) explore the effects of tax–benefit systems on differences in income and incentives to earn income within couples, highlighting important gender differences in effects of taxes and benefits. Figari et al. (2013) describe the redistributive effects of Minimum Income schemes (broadly defined as the ultimate safety net in protecting individuals of working age from poverty) by comparing coverage and adequacy for persons of working age in the European Union.

The Importance of the Tax–Benefit Design   The detailed information provided by a microsimulation model offers the potential for empirical studies focusing on specific design aspects of different tax–benefit instruments. The economic literature has addressed the importance of the channels through which the public intervention characterize a given tax–benefit system. More recently, contributions in behavioral economics point out the importance of the framing effects according to which individuals react, not just to the financial incentives embedded in taxes and benefits but also to the way these are presented (Avram 2015).

Following the emergence of a consensus on the need to have a more simplified tax system and to shift taxes from labor income to less distortionary tax bases, microsimulation models have been used to inform the academic and policy debate on the importance of tax design.

On one hand, different contributions focused on the potential effects of a flat rate income tax, which has become increasingly popular in the policy debate but is limited to Eastern Europe (among others, Paulus and Peichl 2009). On the other hand, the debate has been focused on a revived interest in housing taxation across Europe, focusing on the role played by mortgage interest tax relief (Matsaganis and Flevotomou 2008) and the chances offered to raise tax revenues while lowering the tax wedge on labor income (Figari et al. 2016). Maestri (2013) extends the existing literature by evaluating the redistributive effect of a comprehensive set of housing-related policies, taking into account the tax advantages given to homeowners and the benefits given to individuals renting a house at a rent lower than the market one.

Moreover, indicators based on microsimulation models can capture the importance of tax design when tax and benefit instruments depend directly on the household socio-demographic characteristics, as is the case of the instruments aimed at supporting families with children. Microsimulation models allow researchers to identify the marginal effect of the tax–benefit system due to particular household configurations. For example, Figari et al. (2011b) apply this approach to families with children to calculate "child-contingent" incomes estimated as the change in household disposable income if they did not have children. As shown in Figure 8.2, child-contingent payments (grey bars), capturing not only the transfers but also the tax concessions, account more precisely for the

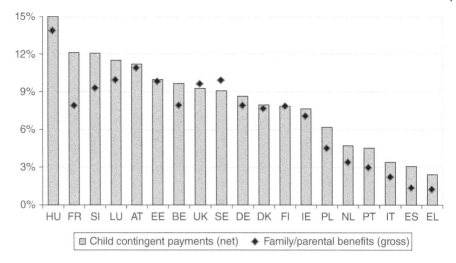

Figure 8.2 Total net child-contingent payments vs. gross family/parental benefits per child as a percentage of per capita disposable income. *Source:* Figari et al. (2011b) using EUROMOD.

full net support provided through tax–benefit systems to families with children compared to gross benefit payments labelled explicitly for children or families (black diamond). The latter is the information typically reported in the survey data.

Another recent example is Salanauskaite and Verbist (2013) who exploit the cross-country comparison to study the role of design characteristics on the public-provided family support in Eastern European countries.

The Economic Downturn: An Opportunity for New Analysis   The economic downturn that has affected the world economy since the end of 2008 reveals the usefulness of the microsimulation approach in providing an ex ante evaluation of the consequences of the crisis on income distribution and social cohesion.

Figari et al. (2011c) and Fernandez Salgado et al. (2014) apply a stress test approach to tax–benefit systems in order to predict the cushioning effects of the social protection schemes for those who lose their jobs and assess the overall income stabilization – through relative and absolute welfare state resilience – after a macroeconomic shock. The stress test approach is borrowed from the analysis of financial institutions where it is used to test the sensitivity of a portfolio to a set of extreme but plausible shocks and assess the significance of the system's vulnerabilities. In context of social policies, the approach uses a microsimulation model to mimic the effects of exogenous shocks (such as a loss of employment or a cut in the salary) on individual and household income.

Callan et al. (2011), Avram et al. (2013), and Paulus et al. (2017) compare the distributional effects of policy changes presented as fiscal consolidation measures in different EU countries that experienced large budget deficits following the financial crisis, highlighting the distributive effects of different policy mixes implemented across Europe. As shown in Figure 8.3, Paulus et al. (2017) estimate the extent to which household income-based austerity measures impact the disposable income of households across European countries most affected by the fiscal consolidation process.

Focusing on Mediterranean countries, Matsaganis and Leventi (2014) distinguish between two inter-related factors: the austerity measures taken to reduce fiscal deficits and the wider recession that hit the economy. They quantify the distributional implications of both factors and provide, in a timely fashion, the first comprehensive assessment of the distributive impact of the crisis in Greece, Italy, Portugal, and Spain.

Dolls et al. (2012) analyze the effectiveness of the tax and transfer systems in the European Union (and the United States) to act as an automatic stabilizer in an economic crisis, showing the extent to which European tax–benefit systems, although heterogeneous, are more effective in absorbing a macroeconomic shock than those in the United States. Moreover, Bargain et al. (2013) show that moving towards a European fiscal union would have a stabilizing effect through either an EU-wide tax and transfer system or an EU-wide system of fiscal equalization.

Beyond Disposable Income: Modeling In-kind Benefits and Indirect Taxes It is widely recognized that economic well-being is a multidimensional concept: income cannot be considered the only indicator of living standards because individual well-being depends also on the economic value of the consumption of goods and of in-kind benefits. The exclusion of consumption expenditure and noncash income from empirical studies of the redistributive effect of tax–benefit systems might also hamper cross-country comparison given the different degree of monetization of the economy across countries. Moreover, the distributional impact of policy changes may be rather different if noncash incomes and indirect taxes are included with important implications for the design of policies aiming to fight poverty and social exclusion, since such an omission may lead to imperfect targeting and misallocation of resources. Given the importance of such aspects, microsimulation models are increasingly including in-kind benefits or indirect taxes within the scope of their analysis.

In-kind benefits, such as services related to child and elderly care, education, health, and public housing, represent about half of welfare state support in European countries and contribute to reducing the inequality otherwise observed in the cash income distribution. The income value of home ownership is another nonmonetary component that enhances the consumption opportunities of

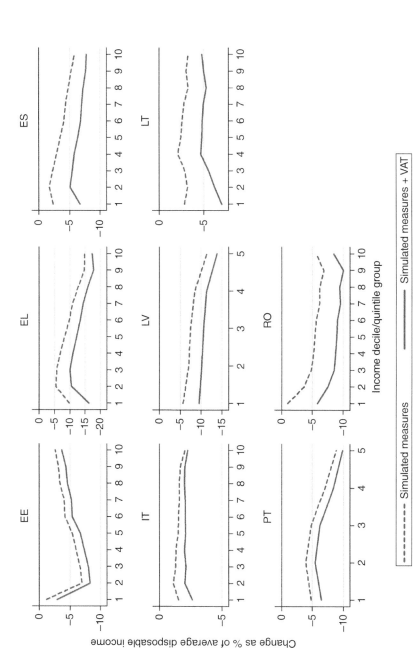

Figure 8.3 Impact of fiscal consolidation measures by household income decile group. *Notes*: Deciles are based on equivalized household disposable income in 2012 in the absence of fiscal consolidation measures and are constructed using the modified OECD equivalence scale. *Source*: Paulus et al. (2017) using EUROMOD.

individuals. The inclusion of in-kind benefits in microsimulation models is becoming more common due to the refinement of different methodological approaches to derive a measure of the value of such benefits (Aaberge et al. 2010a, b; Frick et al. 2010; Paulus et al. 2010).

Indirect taxes (i.e. taxes levied on the exchange value of goods and services) typically represent around 30% of government revenue. While household income surveys used as underlying data for microsimulation models typically do not include detailed information on expenditures, it is nowadays common practice to impute information on expenditures into income surveys and simulate the joint impact on household resources of direct and indirect taxes (Decoster et al. 2010).

Most microsimulation models that include the simulation of indirect taxes rely on the assumption of fixed producer prices (with indirect taxes fully passed to the final price paid by the consumer) and on different assumptions about the behavioral reactions of consumption patterns. To relax these assumptions, one should go beyond a partial equilibrium framework and link the microsimulation models to macro models in order to consider the producer as well as consumer response to specific reforms or economy-wide shocks.

Table 8.2 below shows the incidence of indirect tax payments for three European countries expressed as a percentage of disposable income and as a percentage of

Table 8.2   Incidence of indirect tax payments.

	As % of disposable income			As % of expenditures		
Income decile	Belgium	Greece	UK	Belgium	Greece	UK
1	15.3	37.7	20.2	11.3	13.5	13.9
2	12.0	23.4	13.5	11.8	13.9	14.0
3	11.7	19.8	12.6	12.1	14.3	13.8
4	11.6	18.4	12.4	12.5	14.2	13.8
5	11.4	17.6	11.8	12.7	14.2	14.1
6	11.0	16.0	11.6	12.8	14.1	14.3
7	10.9	16.0	11.1	13.1	14.6	14.5
8	10.8	14.9	10.7	13.3	14.2	14.7
9	10.5	14.2	9.9	13.5	14.3	14.6
10	9.9	11.9	8.2	13.9	14.1	14.4
Total	11.1	16.0	10.8	12.9	14.2	14.3

Notes: Decile groups are formed by ranking individuals according to equivalized household disposable income using the modified OECD equivalence scale
Source: Figari and Paulus (2015) based on EUROMOD.

expenditure, by decile of equivalized disposable income. In the first case (see the left panel of the table) the regressivity of indirect tax payments is clear: poorer individuals pay a larger proportion of their income in indirect taxes compared to richer individuals, mainly due to a larger propensity to consume, and a dissaving behavior that is much more pronounced for the individuals at the bottom of the income distribution whose expenditures, on average, exceed their income (Decoster et al. 2010). In the second case (the right panel of the table), indirect tax payments are progressive and poorer individuals pay a slightly smaller proportion of their total expenditure in VAT and excises compared to richer individuals. The main reason for the lower incidence of indirect taxes at the bottom of the income distribution is that the goods that are VAT exempt or subject to a lower rate (e.g. food, power, domestic fuel, children's clothing) represent a much larger share of total spending of poorer individuals than of richer individuals (Figari and Paulus 2015).

8.3 Microsimulation and the Prediction of Behavioral Changes

The impact of policies on individual behavior through incentives and constraints is at the core of economics. Microsimulation models are valuable tools to provide insights into the potential behavioral reactions to changes in the tax–benefit system and, consequently, into their effects on economic efficiency, income distribution and individual welfare.

A behavioral tax–benefit model is a crucial economic tool for ex ante evaluation of policy reforms to analyze not only the redistributive and fiscal effects but also the behavioral responses of the economic agents in terms of, for example: labor supply, saving, family formation, fertility, location, and mobility. Nevertheless, it is not always necessary to quantify behavioral responses on the assumption that the effects of the policy changes are marginal in relation to the individual budget constraint (Bourguignon and Spadaro 2006), and in some cases, behavior is known to be constrained (e.g. in the case of labor supply adjustments at times of high unemployment). Moreover, behavior takes time to adapt to changing policies, partly because of constraints and lack of information or understanding. This applies most obviously to fertility but also to labor supply in systems where full information on policy rules is not available until the end of the year (after labor supply decisions have already been acted on).

Despite the long tradition in modeling behavior in economics, the most commonly analyzed behavioral reactions to changes in the tax system are only related to labor supply (starting from the seminal contributions of Aaberge et al. (1995) and van Soest (1995)) and programme participation (Keane and Moffitt 1998). The same level of development does not yet apply to other research areas where microsimulation models have been used to investigate, for instance, the potential effects of tax policies on consumption (Creedy 1999; Decoster et al. 2010), savings (Boadway and Wildasin 1995; Feldstein and Feenberg 1983) and housing (King 1983), at least partly due to a lack of suitable data.

Labor Supply Models

There is a general consensus in the literature about using (static) discrete choice models to simulate the individual labor supply reactions to changes in the tax–benefit system. See Aaberge and Colombino (2014) for an extensive review of modeling strategies. Such models, belonging to the family of random utility maximization models, are structural because they provide direct estimations of preferences over income and hours of work through specification of the functional form of the utility function. The discrete choice character of the models is due to the assumption that utility-maximizing individuals and couples choose from a set of a relatively small number alternatives, in terms of working hours, which forms the personal choice set. Each point in the choice set corresponds to a certain disposable income given the gross earnings of each individual (derived using the observed or predicted wage), other incomes, and the tax–benefit system rules simulated by means of a tax–benefit microsimulation model taking into account the socio-demographic characteristics of the family.

In the pre-reform scenario, the labor supply model is estimated on the budget set and provides a direct estimate of the preferences over income and hours. In the post-reform scenario, a new budget set for each family is derived by the tax–benefit model by applying the new tax–benefit rule following the simulated reform. Assuming that the individual random preference heterogeneity as well as the observable preferences do not vary over time, labor supply estimates from the pre-reform scenario are used to predict the labor supply effects and the second round redistributive effects (i.e. when labor supply reactions are taken into account) of the simulated policy reforms.

Recent applications of discrete choice behavioral models are too numerous to be surveyed in this context. Along with many applications focussed on the potential effects of specific tax–benefit policies (among others, see Brewer et al. (2009) for a review of analysis of the effects of in-work benefits across countries), labor supply models based on microsimulation models provide labor supply elasticities that can be used in further tax policy research (Immervoll et al. 2007). Using EUROMOD and TAXSIM, Bargain et al. (2014) provide the first large-scale international comparison of labor supply elasticities including 17 EU countries and the United States. The use of a harmonized approach provides results more robust to possible measurement differences otherwise arising from the use of different

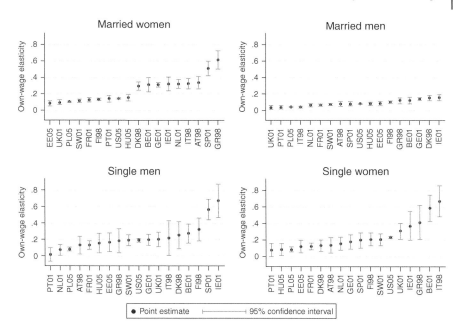

Figure 8.4 Europe and the United States: own-wage elasticities. *Source:* Bargain et al. (2014) using EUROMOD and TAXSIM.

data, microsimulation models and methodological choices. Figure 8.4 shows the estimated own-wage elasticities for single individuals and individuals in couples, which suggest substantial scope for the potential impact of tax–benefit reforms on labor supply and hence income distribution, though the differences across countries are found to be smaller with respect to those in previous studies.

Labor supply estimated preferences and elasticities are a key ingredient in a series of papers on the optimality of tax systems and welfare regimes (Bargain et al. 2011, 2012; Bourguignon and Spadaro 2012; Immervoll et al. 2007, 2011). The cross-country perspective offered by EUROMOD in this context is particularly relevant in order to map the primitive characteristics of the economy (e.g. the inequality in the distribution of the educational attainments) and certain features of the optimal tax–transfer rule (e.g. the degree of progressivity or the type of income support).

Furthermore, Bargain et al. (2014) show the extent to which labor supply elasticities vary with income level with important implications for the analysis of the equity-efficiency trade off inherent in tax–benefit reforms. To this aim, behavioral microsimulation models can be used to implement a computational approach to the optimal taxation problem, allowing the empirical identification of the optimal income tax rules according to various social welfare criteria under the constraint of revenue neutrality (Aaberge and Colombino 2013).

8.4 Beyond Economics: Microsimulation and Other Social Sciences

Microsimulation and Demography

Dynamic microsimulation models extend the time frame of the analysis in order to address the long-term distributional consequences of policy changes, enlarging the perspective of the effects of the policies to individual lifetime and addressing questions about intra-personal redistribution over the lifecycle (Harding 1993). In particular, they are useful tools to analyze, for example, the consequences of different demographic scenarios.

In a long-term perspective, a dynamic microsimulation model aims to capture two main factors. First, the changing structure of the population due to evolving individual and household characteristics (such as age, education, household composition, etc.) and life events (such as marriage, household formation, birth, migration, etc.); second, the interaction of the market mechanisms (e.g. labor market participation, earning levels, etc.) and the tax–benefit system with such characteristics in each point in time.

As clarified in Chapter 7, the aging of individual and household characteristics can be static or dynamic, and the models can be population-based or, more often, focused on specific cohorts of a population (cohort models).

Demographic microsimulation aims to simulate familiar human demographic processes at the individual level. It simulates populations with kinship networks given a set of characteristics of an initial population such as age, sex, marital status, etc. Moreover, to model demographic event decision rules (which may involve more than one individual), a demographic model must specify a stochastic mechanism for adjusting individual heterogeneity, possibly in a heritable way.

In the economics literature, the term "demographic microsimulation" is used to refer to dynamic stochastic microsimulation programs that seek to simulate demographic scenarios and resulting kinship networks (Mason 2014). The output of demographic microsimulation is, therefore, an entire simulated population. Further, microsimulation produces multiple stochastically equivalent realizations of entire populations taking the time factor into consideration. This advantage makes the microsimulation method a very useful tool compared to static models (which do not account for time) and deterministic models (which provide only one outcome).

As clarified above, demographic microsimulations can be identified as agent-based models if their objective is to use macro-regularities or observed data to determine whether ethnographically reasonable rules might be applied (Hammel and Wachter 1996). Alternatively, demographic microsimulations used to test consistency of rules themselves with macroscopic Bayesian priors are also considered to be agent-based models (Zagheni 2011).

There are, however, some applications of demographic microsimulation that do not fit comfortably with the common concept of an agent-based model. In some studies, researchers set exogenously and validate externally the value of some demographic variables of interest in order to explore the implications of assumed demographic rate. Although in these microsimulations the "agent" (population) acts independently, the method used substantially differs from the known agent-based methodology.

Applications

There are four main overlapping areas of study where demographic microsimulation models are used to test and quantify the effects of changes in kin networks: (i) long-term changes in fertility and mortality; (ii) rule, policies, and preferences; (iii) HIV/AIDS; (iv) methods of estimating demographic quantities.

Long-term changes in fertility and mortality, such as in the aging population, future low fertility rate, etc., can be stated only under stable population assumptions. This assumption holds in the long run if the entire distribution is known. Demographic microsimulations provide researchers with this information. By using demographic simulations, many studies estimate kinship resources in order to investigate long-term changes in fertility and mortality, for example their decline in China (Hammel et al. 1991; Lin 1994, 1995; Zhao 1998), population aging in the United States (Smith 1991), and the effects of demographic transitions in England (Lesthaeghe 1995; Murphy 2010, 2011).

Rules and preferences toward behavior have implications on demographic events and kinship networks. It is hard to analytically model a complex order of individual preferences. Microsimulation models can simulate behavioral responses of a large set of kin, even for those who may not exist at certain ages at a given point in time. Preferences toward and prohibitions on marriage between certain types of kin, individual and societal preferences for extended families, and patterns of marriage deeply affect kinship networks that can be hypothetically reproduced by demographic microsimulations. For example, Hammel et al. (1979) investigate delayed marriage as a cause of fertility loss and its relationship to kinship resources. Ruggles (1987) analyses kinship networks in rich historical contexts to show that changing demography was a necessary but not a sufficient condition for increasing the number of extended families. Murphy (2011) studies the changing patterns of marriage and their effects on England's kinship networks. In his work, Wachter (1997) microsimulates immigration, birth, death, marriage, and divorce in the United States to explain, similarly to Bartlema (1988), how serial monogamy affects the frequency of step-kin.

Demographic changes in kinship resources and networks are dramatically driven by diseases. Especially in poor countries, viruses such as HIV create enormous financial, emotional, and opportunity costs of caring for family members that are difficult to measure with traditional demographic techniques. Wachter et al. (2002), Zagheni (2011), and Sevcikova et al. (2007) use microsimulations to quantify the presence of HIV on burden of care, on orphanhood and infection rates.

Many studies apply demographic microsimulations seeking to estimate demographic quantities in scenarios of poor or imperfect information (Goldman 1978; Goodman et al. 1974; Hammel and Wachter 1996). Finally, microsimulation models appear to be a powerful tool to test research assumptions and violation of them. Wachter (1980) and McDaniel and Hammel (1984) develop new measures for population growth and measure their performance under different (more realistic) assumptions.

8.5   Microsimulation and Geography

Spatial Models

Geographical information on household income, wealth, taxation, welfare benefit, and in general, on the welfare state of a region are essential for policy makers. In recent years, researchers have developed spatial indicators useful for policy formulation and implementation; however, there is a lack of geographical data on household behavior especially for small areas. Most countries use a Census to derive small area social and demographic data, but a Census is expensive and usually not conducted every year. The importance of using updated information in the policymaking process has motivated researchers to develop spatial microsimulation models (Tanton 2014), as clarified in Chapter 7.

As for tax–benefit microsimulation models, spatial models can be classified into static and dynamic models. Static microsimulation models can calculate variables of interest in different what-if scenarios using the base dataset, but they cannot model life events. On the other hand, dynamic microsimulation models take a base dataset and model life events, like marriages and deaths, along a time framework for a specific spatial unit.

Micro Data Generation: Synthetic Reconstruction Versus Reweighting

Most of the spatial microsimulation models use known aggregates coming from Census and/or administrative data as benchmarks. They include information such as age, sex, family characteristics, employment status, incomes, rent payments, education, housing, etc. These known aggregates are necessary in order to create unit record files for each small area when using a static spatial microsimulation model. Spatial static microsimulation methods can be divided into two groups: synthetic reconstruction methods and reweighting approaches.

Reweighting approaches reweight already available surveys or sample datasets to known small area characteristics (Tanton 2014). There are different methods that use a reweighting approach. One method is the combinatorial optimization (CO) which selects observations from a survey until some known benchmark totals are reached. For example, it can select a set of households from microdata to reproduce, as closely as possible, the population in the small area. This is an iterative method that starts with a random selection and keeps replacing the observation until a certain goodness-of-fit is achieved. Another method which uses a reweighting approach is quota sampling. In contrast to the CO method, quota sampling uses sampling without replacement, thus consistently improves computational efficiency. A very common method which uses a reweighting approach is the generalized regression procedure (Tanton et al. 2011, 2013). It reweights survey data in order to aggregate reliable data and uses regression models to calculate a new set of weights given the constraints for each small area. The generalized regression procedure is an iterative process: it takes an initial weight from the survey and adjusts this weight until a target result is achieved or the number of possible iterations is reached. There are many applications of this method for estimating poverty (Tanton et al. 2011; Tanton et al. 2010), wealth (Vidyattama et al. 2013), and disability (Lymer et al. 2008, 2009).

Applications

Spatial microsimulation models can have substantial impact on public policy because they provide policymakers with indicators of income, poverty rates, and subjective well-being (Anderson 2007) of different geographic areas. Moreover, they allow policymakers to obtain information on the spatial effects of policy changes (Ballas et al. 2005b; O'Donoghue et al. 2012; Tanton et al. 2010). Spatial microsimulation models have, in fact, many applications. Mainly, researchers used them to derive estimates of characteristics of small areas: income (Anderson 2007) crime (Kongmuang et al. 2006), poverty (Tanton et al. 2011; Tanton et al. 2010), obesity (Edwards and Clarke 2012; Procter et al. 2008), water demand (Clarke et al. 1997; Williamson et al. 1996), smoking rates (Smith et al. 2011; Tomintz et al. 2008, 2009), wellbeing (Ballas 2010; Mohanty et al. 2013), disability (Lymer et al. 2008), etc. Combining together microsimulation models is common in the literature and spatial microsimulation models are often combined with a tax/transfer microsimulation model to estimate effects of policy changes. For example, Harding et al. (2009) examine the national and local impacts of a possible family-oriented tax benefit reform in Australia; Tanton et al. (2010) estimate the change in poverty rates due to policy changes affecting elderly people in Australia; Vu and Tanton (2010) analyze the distributional and regional impact of the Australian Government's Household Stimulus Package. Tomintz et al. (2008)

and Tomintz et al. (2013) link a spatial simulation model to location-allocation models to help locate health care facilities. Herault (2007) and Buddelmeyer et al. (2012) link spatial microsimulation models to CGE models to derive small area impacts of macroeconomic changes. Recently, spatial microsimulation models are often used to make socio-demographic projections. Methods for projecting births, deaths, and migration using static ageing are described in Vidyattama and Tanton (2010, 2013) whereas examples of applications are in Ballas et al. (2005a, b).

8.6 Microsimulation and Transports

Characterization of Space, Mode and Time

As mentioned in the Introduction, transport-related research is an area in which the combination of agent-based and microsimulation models has proved its potential, and the literature is not always clear on the overlapping of and distinctions between different modeling approaches. Nevertheless, a modeling-based approach is nowadays a mainstream tool for analyzing a variety of transportation phenomena, including transportation network operations (both road and transit) and travel demand forecasting. Microsimulation models and data driven agent-based models are used for hypotheses testing and experimentation with alternative models of travel behavior, and for operational planning, design, and system control.

Microsimulation of transportation systems is challenging given its high dimensionality in space (travel from various origins to various destinations along many routes and modes of travel), time (frequency of travel), and characteristics of those who make the trip or, in case of freight, type of shipment. Generally, transportation models are classified according to the spatial context being modeled (urban versus interregional travel) or according to the object of travel (person or freight/goods).

Freight transportation microsimulation models have found somehow limited interest so far between researchers (Boerkamps et al. 2000; Fischer et al. 2005). Person travel models have not generally been the focus of microsimulation modeling, although the microsimulation components of these models are the same as those used in urban modeling applications. The latter applications have been developed since the mid-1950s in North America and Europe (Meyer and Miller 2001).

In urban microsimulation models, the basic unit of travel is the trip: a movement from a single origin to a single destination at a given time by a given travel mode via a given route through the transportation network. The trip is not an action per se, but it is made in order to engage in an activity at the trip destination.

These concepts are applied in the standard paradigm for modeling trip-making in urban areas, known as the Urban Transportation Modeling System (UTMS), or, more commonly, the "four-step" model.

The four-step model predicts the travel demand in four steps: (i) determination of the number of trips generated within the urban region (Trip generation); (ii) spatial distribution of trip destinations (Trip distribution); (iii) travel mode for each trip (Mode split); (iv) route from origin to destination through the transit network used by each trip, given the spatial population distribution and the transportation system serving the local demand (Trip assignment). The four-step model is spatially aggregate, its unit of analysis is the origin-destination trip flows rather than individual trips, and it is static, meaning that time does not enter in the model system. Thus, the total trips are generated for a given time period according to a path-independent static equilibrium system state.

Because of its aggregate nature, the four-step process does not capture the heterogeneity of the trip-making behavior and the nonlinear form of the trip-makers' decision function. Therefore, the model generates bias aggregate parameters. Moreover, the static nature of the four-step model does not consider factors such as road traffic, transit operations, atmospheric emissions, and time-dependent elements of travel demand (timing of trip, etc.). To avoid bias in the travel predictions and to model travelling behavior within and over time, researchers have to disaggregate data and estimate the model parameters in a disaggregate way (per each individual trip-maker).

Dynamic microsimulation models can predict travel demands in terms of number of trips occurring within a large urban region, by purpose, by time of day, by origin and destination, and by mode, dealing with spatial, temporal and socio-economic and demographic heterogeneity. The following section discusses these models in more detail.

Travel Demand, Route Choice and Network Performance

Dynamic microsimulation models can be categorized into (i) travel demand models, and (ii) route choice and network performance simulation models. These models use quite different methods and are implemented with separate software packages, thus creating separate research areas.

Travel demand microsimulation models share common concepts and assumptions. For example, travel is considered to be a derived demand: people travel in order to reach a precise destination and/or to engage in a specific activity. Therefore, an activity-based approach is implemented to estimate a daily activity pattern, which includes information on timing and destination of trips, modes of travel, etc. In travel demand models, time and space are constraints as are other individuals' attributes like income, possible use of car, lack of driving licence, etc.

Agents in these models are trip-makers who choose their activity patterns and associated travel such that their individual utility is maximized.

The Random Utility Maximization (RUM) model is the most common model which assumes that decision-makers are rational utility maximizers; in other words, they choose an alternative within a set of feasible alternatives which maximizes their utility. In addition to RUM-based models, researchers can opt for rule or Computational Process Models (CPMs) that employ nonRUM decision rules, like elimination-by-aspect rule (Ben-Akiva and Bierlaire 1999; Recker and Golob 1979; Tversky 1972) and bounded rationality/satisficing approach (Fujii and Garling 2003; Kitamura and Fujii 1998; Simon 1957; Williams and Ortuzar 1982).

Travel demand microsimulation models can also be classified according to a methodological approach into tour-based models and activity scheduling models. Tour-based models focus on choosing a daily set of trips for each person where trips consist of one or more tours. These models provide the simulation of a daily travel for each person in the region generated by sequential decisions that pursue objectives of time, destination, mode, and route for each trip of the tour. Activity scheduling models, on the contrary, focus more directly on modeling actual activity patterns. According to this approach, trips are generated to move each person from an activity location to another. It is only in the second step of the process that the travel mode and route choice are determined.

In microsimulating route choice and network performance, researchers use separate models according to the type of network: road, transit, and walk (or bicycle). These are quite different networks since both the path choice and the vehicle/person movement are very different.

The most developed network models with a very large research community and resources are the road network models. Their aim is to simulate vehicle movements through a network where travel demand and paths from origin to destination are fixed. Because these models are computationally demanding, they are usually used for the analysis of a specific network segment. These models are very powerful: they replicate traffic flow behavior very well. Some of the road network models look at the route choice as a dynamic equilibrium problem in which each driver attempts to find the minimum time path through the network for her/his trip. In these models – called mesoscopic DTA models – equilibrium occurs when no driver can unilaterally change paths through the network and improve her/his travel time. Essential for these models is the definition of path time, which can be either calculated before the trip starts or experienced along the network links that are actually involved in the trip.

Transit network modeling is more complicated to implement since many factors involved in the network are difficult to measure, such as comfort, reliability, and security. The transit path choice depends also on many variables, such as wait and transfer times, fares, etc., which are complex variables to estimate. Interestingly, pedestrian and bicycle modeling is not very well developed. Given the large number of pedestrians, these models are very computationally demanding. However, some approaches to microsimulating pedestrian and bicycle movements are used (Bandini et al. 2007; Blue and Adler 2001; Robin 2011; Sahaleh et al. 2012; Zhang et al. 2013), including the modeling of mixed auto and bicycle flows (Dijkstra 2012; Vasic and Ruskin 2011). It is not surprising that increased attention will be paid in the future to the development of these types of models because of the growing importance of bicycling in many urban areas.

Applications

A clear example of a travel demand microsimulation model that uses a computational process approach is ALBATROSS (Arentze and Timmermans 2000, 2004). It is an operational model which determines the activity schedule for a given day for a given trip-maker, given a set of trip-maker attributes. The activity schedule decision is statistically derived from observed activity/travel data using the CHIAD method (Kass 1980) that divides trip-makers into homogenous groups with respect to a decision variable (e.g. travel mode) given a set of constraints. CHIAD maximizes a Chi-square measure of dissimilarity between groups (Arentze and Timmermans 2004).

An example of a tour-based travel demand microsimulation model is ARC (Atlanta Regional Commission). ARC determines the final location, the type of daily activity pattern, and the number of tours (frequency) in a day for each of the trip-makers. Costs, road and transit networks are specified for each tour. Contrary to ARC, TASHA – the Canadian Travel/Activity Scheduler for Household Agents – is a travel demand microsimulation model which uses an activity scheduling approach (Miller and Roorda 2003; Roorda et al. 2008). TASHA determines the number and duration of individual activity by type of activity and involves a Monte Carlo draws from empirical probability frequency distributions of activities and sequentially generates activity episodes scheduled for each trip-maker.

Two road models (belonging to the route choice and network performance category) that are widely cited in the travel microsimulation literature are TRANSIMS and MATSim. They have been specifically designed to be computationally efficient in the simulation of road choices in large urban regions. They are full travel demand and network modeling systems; this means they are not just limited to the simulation of the route path through the transit network. Moreover, they are fully agent-based models in which the movements of individuals are modeled in a multi-modal setting.

8.7   Microsimulation and Environmental Sciences

Scope and Spatial Disaggregation

Over the past years, environmental issues have dramatically grown in importance alongside the desire to find effective solutions and create appropriate public policies. Environmental policies such as regulations, carbon taxes, and emissions trading require an ex ante analysis and impact assessment. Microsimulation models are particularly useful for this type of investigation because they can carry out complex simulations of possible strategies to be applied and evaluate the consequences on the local economy.

A key feature of environmental and natural resources economics is represented by the interaction between human activity and the environment, which is strongly influenced by spatial location. Spatial dimensions characterize environmental microsimulation models. These dimensions can be divided into the spatial scope and spatial disaggregation of the model. The spatial scope can vary from a village to a city, from a country to a continent. The relevant scope depends on user objectives. Spatial disaggregation refers to the spatial levels within models. For example, the size of the unit of analysis can decrease from a country to a region to a local area. The greater the degree of spatial disaggregation, the greater the degree of inter-area analysis that is conducted (Minot and Baulch 2005).

Spatial disaggregation tends to be on the district or zone level, although many microsimulation models such as agri-environmental models utilize a national level unit of analysis (Hynes et al. 2009a, b). Benenson (2007) claims that the chosen level of disaggregation may affect investigation conclusions. It has been shown, for example, that the impact of pollutants is nonlinear related to spatial concentration. This means that a low level of disaggregation may underestimate the significance of the impact. However, in many cases, it is not possible to apply a high level of disaggregation because data is not available (Felsenstein et al. 2010).

Scope and spatial disaggregation are also important for the valuation of environmental goods and services. Bateman et al. (2006) argue that the market for environmental goods may be a more significant determinant of the aggregate value placed on a specific good than the average value that an individual holds for that good. Moreover, they show that the political jurisdiction often used in aggregating environmental value estimates is usually larger than the economic jurisdiction. The latter is the group of individuals that are actually involved in a specific policy. In this way, any type of analysis that does not acknowledge this spatial inconsistency would produce biased results.

Modeling Pollution and Natural Resources

Environmental microsimulation models are based on microdata; therefore, in modeling pollution, the first step is to generate data if not available. Usually, polluting behavior is expressed in value terms; for example, the amount of fuel or energy consumed. Microsimulation models thus generate the volumes of use (O'Donoghue 1997). The next step is to model the amount of pollution generated associated with specific volumes. It is common, for example, to model greenhouse gas emissions using carbon parameters (Chakraborty et al. 2006; McQuinn and Binfield 2002).

Microsimulation models are also used to analyze the impact of changes in environmental policies and provide examples of modeling of marginal costs of abatement. For example, Doole (2012) is interested in the nitrogen marginal cost of abatement curve at farm level, while Dieckhoener and Hecking (2012) model the greenhouse gas abatement cost curve in relation to residential heating markets.

The Valuation of Nonmarket Public Goods and Benefit Transfers

Modeling the spatial incidence of the environmental issues (pollution, etc.) or the behavioral impact of environmental policies is the main focus of environmental microsimulation models. However, micro-data environmental simulation methods have also been used for the calculation of welfare measures for environmental goods that are not generally traded in an established market (nonmarket goods). Thus, researchers use microsimulation for the estimation of the so-called valuation models (usually discrete choice models) that provide estimates of the nonmarket value of environmental benefits. A possible approach in these models is the Benefit Transfers (BTs) approach (Johnston and Rosenberger 2010) which utilizes the results related to studies on a wide range of environmental goods and services to create a sort of benchmark for an environmental analysis. This method has the advantage of yielding important information in many scientific and management contexts used as a meaningful basis for the application of environmental policies (Brouwer 2000; Ledoux and Turner 2002; Rosenberger and Loomis 2001).

The BTs approach has been used in the implementation of environmental policies such as the EU Water Framework Directive (Hanley et al. 2006), health risks associated with water quality (Kask and Shogren 1994), air quality (Rozan 2004), and forest management (Bateman et al. 2006). Alberini and Scarpa (2005) provide a review of the studies that make use of microsimulation methods for environmental valuation.

Socioeconomic and Environmental Interactions

Environmental microsimulation models have to take into account the interactions between the environment and the socioeconomic aspects of an area. Sometimes, the aim of a microsimulation model is modeling of the socio-economic-environmental interactions and policies themselves (Hynes and O'Donoghue 2014). Many studies in the literature have focussed on these macro–micro linkages (Hérault, et al., 2009). It is common between researchers to link a microsimulation model to an input–output model. The input–output methodology (Leontief 1951) provides information about sectors of an economy, pointing out the input flows from one sector to another (or directly to the final demand). Outputs in the model can either be final outputs for the final demand or they can be inputs for other sectors. With this model, it is possible to get a distributional estimate of the direct environmental impacts or policies, and to measure an indirect effect related to behavioral responses (for example the consumption of other goods or services).

A very recent application of models that explore the socioeconomic–environmental interactions is by Boccanfuso et al. (2013). Authors simulate the diminishing productivity of agricultural land as a consequence of climate change for Senegal and analyze the impact of climate change policies introduced to reduce greenhouse gas emissions. They find that decreases in land productivity together with increasing world fossil fuel price have a negative impact on poverty. Moreover, they claim that subsidising electricity consumption to protect households from fuel price increases does not substantially improve the poverty situation of an economy.

Applications

Environmental microsimulation models have mainly been used to simulate natural resources demand and environmental issues, and to analyze the distributional incidence of environmental policies. In this section we provide some examples.

Regarding the environmental problems and natural resources demand and management, we find many studies in the literature. For example, Barton et al. (2000) and Sander et al. (2009) develop a spatial microsimulation model for disaster simulations. Brouwers (2005) and Brouwers and Linnerooth-Bayer (2003) simulate the spatial impact of flooding-related disasters. Smith and Strauss (1986) use a spatial microsimulation method to model a subsistence environment in Sierra Leone. Dijk et al. (1996) develop a microsimulation model to analyze the nutrient flow approach for Dutch agriculture. In regard to greenhouse gas emissions, many simulations have been carried out (Hynes et al. 2009b, 2013;

Lal and Follett 2009). Many researchers are interested in forecasting water demand (Clarke et al. 1997; Mitchell 1999; Williamson 2001; Williamson et al. 2002). Complex models that involve natural resources usage and environmental impacts in a unique framework have also been created. CitySim (Robinson et al. 2009) simulates at the micro level the impact of energy use, transportation, and waste management on environmental sustainability. Noth et al. (2003) developed UrbanSim to simulate the development of urban areas including land use, transportation, and environmental impacts over periods of time.

There is an extensive body of literature on modeling the distributive impacts of environmental policies. Distributional implications of environmental taxes have been explored by O'Donoghue (1997), Callan et al. (2009), Hamilton and Cameron (1994), Labandeira and Labeaga (1999), Labandeira et al. (2007), Bureau (2011), Casler and Rafiqui (1993), Symons et al. (1994), Yusuf (2008), Bach et al. (2002), Bork (2006), Cornwell and Creedy (1996), and Buddelmeyer et al. (2012).

Environmental policies such as tradable emissions have been assessed using microsimulation models by Waduda et al. (2008) while taxes on nitrogen emissions have been analyzed by Berntsen et al. (2003). Simulations of "what-if" scenarios such as the impact of changes in consumptions on emissions have been carried out by Alfredsson (2004). Research on climate change impact simulations is dramatically increasing. For instance, Breisinger et al. (2011) and Bussolo et al. (2008) study the effects of weather changes on food security.

8.8 Conclusions

Microsimulation modeling is employed to analyze the interactions between policies and the complexities of economic and social life, as well as the interactions between policies of different types. For example, microsimulation techniques are widely applied for the analysis of tax–benefit policies, of different demographic scenarios, of life events such as births and migration in different geographical areas, and of transport choices. This chapter provides an overview of various applications of microsimulation models in social sciences that enormously increased in the recent decades. Specifically, the chapter reviews some important microsimulation approaches in economics, demography, geography, transport, and environmental sciences, while identifying potential overlaps among research areas.

Microsimulation models are widely used in applied public economics and quantitative social sciences. They are very powerful tools in calculating the effects of a given policy on the distribution of household income and its components. Moreover, through the simulation of counterfactual scenarios, they deliver the information on the effects of alternative policy regimes. Any policy change brings financing and budgetary consequences together with redistributive income effects, which can be explored by using microsimulation techniques. Finally, microsimulation investigations quantify the impact of tax–benefit programmes on behavioral responses in terms of, for example, labor supply, saving, fertility, location, and mobility. Behavioral microsimulation models offer evidence that substantially contribute to the policy debate on the importance of tax design. Overall, the microsimulation approach in economics provides ex ante evaluation of possible consequences of micro and macro-economic shocks on the well-being of individuals.

Similarly, microsimulation models are implemented in order to measure the consequences of different demographic scenarios. The population structure continuously evolves because of household characteristics and life events. Therefore, researchers in this area find very useful a dynamic microsimulation approach, which allows quantifying the effects of changes in kin networks while accounting for time. Demographic microsimulations seek to estimate demographic quantities even in the case of imperfect information.

Incomplete information is a common issue for spatial models. Very often, a lack of geographical data, especially for small areas, implies some difficulties in the prediction of household behavior. The need of informing the policy maker incentivized the use of dynamic microsimulation models suitable to simulate life events, like marriage and deaths, along the time framework for a specific location. Spatial microsimulations calculate indicators of many characteristics of specific geographic areas: income, crime, poverty, well-being, etc. that are particularly useful in the formulation and evaluation of public policies.

One of the main applications of microsimulation models refers to transport-related research. The travel demand can be estimated by considering the travel modes, the possible destinations, the frequency of travel, and the characteristics of the users. Transport microsimulation applications (and spatial applications) can overlap with microsimulation applications in environmental sciences because of the key feature of the interactions between human activities and the environment. Environmental issues (e.g. pollution) require effective public policies. It became crucial and convenient the use of microsimulations based on microdata that can generate data not available. The spatial incidence of the environmental policies are hence provided together with the impact on socioeconomic aspects.

Microsimulations in social sciences clearly allow researchers to carry out social-economic investigations that significantly support the policy-making processes by estimating the impact of different public policies in counterfactual scenarios. The policy maker is therefore better informed on the potential consequences of governmental decisions on the variables of interest and ultimately can choose the optimal policy design for a specific group of population.

References

Aaberge, R. and Colombino, U. (2013). Designing optimal taxes with a microeconometric model of household labor supply. *Scandinavian Journal of Economics* 115 (2): 449–475.

Aaberge, R. and Colombino, U. (2014). Microsimulation and labor supply models: a survey and an interpretation. In: *Handbook of Microsimulation* (ed. C. O'Donogue), 167–221. Bingley: Emerald.

Aaberge, R., Dagsvik, J.K., and Strøm, S. (1995). Labor supply responses and welfare effects of tax reforms. *Scandinavian Journal of Economics* 97 (4): 635–659.

Aaberge, R., Bhuller, M., Langørgen, A., and Mogstad, M. (2010a). The distributional impact of public services when needs differ. *Journal of Public Economics* 94 (9–10): 549–562.

Aaberge, R., Langørgen, A., and Lindgren, P. (2010b). The impact of basic public services on the distribution of income in European countries. In: *Income and Living Conditions in Europe* (eds. A.B. Atkinson and E. Marlier), 329–344. Luxembourg: Eurostat Statistical Books, Publications Office of the European Union (Chapter 15).

Alberini, A. and Scarpa, R. (eds.) (2005). *Applications of Simulation Methods in Environmental and Resource Economics*, 29–36. Dordrecht: Springer.

Alfredsson, E.C. (2004). "Green" consumption – no solution for climate change. *Energy* 29 (4): 513–524.

Anderson, B. (2007). *Creating Small-area Income Estimates: Spatial Microsimulation Modeling*. UK Department of Communities.

Arentze, T. and Timmermans, H. (2000). *Albatross: A Learning Based Transportation Oriented Simulation System*. Eindhoven: Eirass.

Arentze, T.A. and Timmermans, H.J. (2004). A learning-based transportation oriented simulation system. *Transportation Research Part B: Methodological* 38 (7): 613–633.

Avram, S. (2015). Benefit losses loom larger than taxes: the effects of framing and loss aversion on behavioural responses to taxes and benefits. ISER working paper series 2015-17.

Avram, S., Figari, F., Leventi, C. et al. (2013). The distributional effects of fiscal consolidation in nine EU countries. EUROMOD working paper EM2/13, University of Essex.

Bach, S., Kohlhaas, M., Meyer, B. et al. (2002). The effects of environmental fiscal reform in Germany: a simulation study. *Energy Policy* 30 (9): 803–811.

Ballas, D. (2010). Geographical modeling of happiness and well-being. In: *Spatial and Social Disparities* (eds. J. Stillwell, P. Norman, C. Thomas and P. Surridge), 53–66. The Netherlands: Springer.

Ballas, D., Clarke, G., Dorling, D. et al. (2005a). SimBritain: a spatial microsimulation approach to population dynamics. *Population, Space and Place* 11 (1): 13–34.

Ballas, D., Rossiter, D., Thomas, B. et al. (2005b). *Geography Matters: Simulating the Local Impacts of National Social Policies.* New York: Joseph Rowntree Foundation.

Bandini, S., Federici, M.L., and Vizzari, G. (2007). Situated cellular agents approach to crowd modeling and simulation. *Cybernetics and Systems: An International Journal* 38 (7): 729–753.

Bargain, O. (2012a). Decomposition analysis of distributive policies using behavioural simulations. *International Tax and Public Finance* 19 (5): 708–731.

Bargain, O. (2012b). The distributional effects of tax-benefit policies under New Labor: a decomposition approach. *Oxford Bulletin of Economics and Statistics* 74 (6): 856–874.

Bargain, O. and Callan, T. (2010). Analysing the effects of tax-benefit reforms on income distribution: a decomposition approach. *Journal of Economic Inequality* 8 (1): 1–21.

Bargain O., Dolls M., Neumann D. et al. (2011). Tax-benefit systems in Europe and the US: between equity and efficiency. IZA discussion paper 5440.

Bargain, O., Decoster, A., Dolls, M. et al. (2012). Welfare, labor supply and heterogeneous preferences: evidence for Europe and the US. *Social Choice and Welfare* 41: 789–817.

Bargain, O., Dolls, M., Fuest, C. et al. (2013). Fiscal union in Europe? Redistributive and stabilizing effects of a European tax-benefit system and fiscal equalization mechanism. *Economic Policy* 28 (75): 375–422.

Bargain, O., Orsini, K., and Peichl, A. (2014). Comparing labor supply elasticities in Europe and the US: new results. *Journal of Human Resources* 49 (3): 723–838.

Bartlema, J. (1988). Modeling step-families. *European Journal of Population/Revue Européenne de Démographie* 4 (3): 197–221.

Barton, D.C., Eidson, E.D., Schoenwald, D.A. et al. (2000). *Aspen-ee: An Agent-Based Model of Infrastructure Interdependency. SAND2000-2925.* Albuquerque, NM: Sandia National Laboratories.

Bateman, I.J., Day, B.H., Georgiou, S., and Lake, I. (2006). The aggregation of environmental benefit values: welfare measures, distance decay and total WTP. *Ecological Economics* 60 (2): 450–460.

Ben-Akiva, M. and Bierlaire, M. (1999). Discrete choice methods and their applications to short term travel decisions. In: *Handbook of Transportation Science* (ed. R.W. Hall), 5–33. US: Springer.

Benenson, I. (2007). Warning! The scale of land-use CA is changing! Computers. *Environment and Urban Systems* 31 (2): 107–113.

Berntsen, J., Petersen, B.M., Jacobsen, B.H. et al. (2003). Evaluating nitrogen taxation scenarios using the dynamic whole farm simulation model FASSET. *Agricultural Systems* 76 (3): 817–839.

Billari, F.C., Ongaro, F., and Prskawetz, A. (2003). *Introduction: Agent-Based Computational Demography*, 1–17. Physica-Verlag HD.

Blue, V.J. and Adler, J.L. (2001). Cellular automata microsimulation for modeling bi-directional pedestrian walkways. *Transportation Research Part B: Methodological* 35 (3): 293–312.

Blundell, R. (2012). Tax policy reform: the role of empirical evidence. *Journal of the European Economic Association* 10 (1): 43–77.

Blundell, R. and Shepard, A. (2012). Employment, hours of work and the optimal taxation of low income families. *Review of Economic Studies* 79: 481–510.

Boadway, R. and Wildasin, D. (1995). Taxation and savings: a survey. *Fiscal Studies* 15 (3): 19–63.

Boccanfuso, D., Savard, L., and Estache, A. (2013). The distributional impact of developed countries' climate change policies on Senegal: a macro-micro CGE application. *Sustainability* 5 (6): 2727–2750.

Boerkamps, J., van Binsbergen, A., and Bovy, P. (2000). Modeling behavioral aspects of urban freight movement in supply chains. *Transportation Research Record: Journal of the Transportation Research Board* 1725: 17–25.

Borella, M. and Coda Moscarola, F. (2010). Microsimulation of pension reforms: behavioural versus non behavioural approach. *Journal of Pension Economics and Finance* 9 (4): 583–607.

Bork, C. (2006). Distributional effects of the ecological tax reform in Germany: an evaluation with a microsimulation model. In: *The Distributional Effects of Environmental Policy* (eds. Y. Serret and N. Johnstone), 139–170. Northampton, MA: Edward Elgar Publishing.

Bourguignon, F. and Bussolo, M. (2013). Income distribution in computable general equilibrium modeling. In: *Handbook of Computable General Equilibrium Modeling*, Volume 1A and 1B, Chapter 21 (eds. P.B. Dixon and D.W. Jorgenson), 1383–1437. Elsevier.

Bourguignon, F. and Spadaro, A. (2006). Microsimulation as a tool for evaluating redistribution policies. *Journal of Economic Inequality* 4 (1): 77–106.

Bourguignon, F. and Spadaro, A. (2012). Tax–benefit revealed social preferences. *Journal of Economic Inequality* 10 (1): 75–108.

Breisinger, C., Ecker, O., Al-Riffai, P. et al. (2011). Climate change, agricultural production and food security: evidence from Yemen (No. 1747). Kiel working papers.

Brewer, M., Francesconi, M., Gregg, P., and Grogger, J. (2009). In-work benefit reform in a cross-national perspective – introduction. *The Economic Journal* 119 (535): F1–F14.

Brouwer, R. (2000). Environmental value transfer: state of the art and future prospects. *Ecological Economics* 32 (1): 137–152.

Brouwers, L. (2005). Microsimulation models for disaster policy making. Doctoral dissertation. Stockholm.

Brouwers, L. and Linnerooth-Bayer, J. (2003). Spatial and Dynamic Modeling of Flood Management Policies in the Upper Tisza. *Interim Report IR-03-02*. International Institute for Applied Systems Analysis (IIASA), Laxenburg, Austria.

Buddelmeyer, H., Hérault, N., Kalb, G., and de Jong, M.V.Z. (2012). Linking a microsimulation model to a dynamic CGE model: climate change mitigation policies and income distribution in Australia. *International Journal of Microsimulation* 5 (2): 40–58.

Bureau, B. (2011). Distributional effects of a carbon tax on car fuels in France. *Energy Economics* 33 (1): 121–130.

Bussolo, M., de Hoyos, R., Medvedev, D., and van der Mensbrugghe, D. (2008). *Global Climate Change and Its Distributional Impacts.* Washington, DC: World Bank.

Callan, T., Lyons, S., Scott, S. et al. (2009). The distributional implications of a carbon tax in Ireland. *Energy Policy* 37 (2): 407–412.

Callan T., Leventi, C., Levy, H. et al. (2011). The distributional effects of austerity measures: a comparison of six EU countries. EUROMOD working paper series EM6/11.

Casler, S.D. and Rafiqui, A. (1993). Evaluating fuel tax equity: direct and indirect distributional effects. *National Tax Journal* 46 (2): 197–205.

Chakraborty, A., Bhattacharya, D.K., and Li, B.L. (2006). Spatiotemporal dynamics of methane emission from rice fields at global scale. *Ecological complexity* 3 (3): 231–240.

Cingano, F. and Faiella, I. (2013). Green taxation in Italy: an assessment of a carbon tax on transport. Bank of Italy Occasional Paper No. 206.

Clarke, G.P., Kashti, A., McDonald, A., and Williamson, P. (1997). Estimating small area demand for water: a new methodology. *Water and Environment Journal* 11 (3): 186–192.

Cornwell, A. and Creedy, J. (1996). Carbon taxation, prices and inequality in Australia. *Fiscal Studies* 17 (3): 21–38.

Creedy, J. (1999). *Modeling Indirect Taxes and Tax Reform.* Northampton, MA: Edward Elgar.

Decoster, A., Loughrey, J., O'Donoghue, C., and Verwerft, D. (2010). How regressive are indirect taxes? A microsimulation analysis for five European countries. *Journal of Policy Analysis & Management* 29 (2): 326–350.

Dieckhoener, C. and Hecking, H. (2012). Greenhouse gas abatement cost curves of the residential heating market–a microeconomic approach (No. 12/16). EWI working paper.

Dijk, J., Leneman, H., and van der Veen, M. (1996). The nutrient flow model for Dutch agriculture: a tool for environmental policy evaluation. *Journal of Environmental Management* 46 (1): 43–55.

Dolls, M., Fuest, C., and Peichl, A. (2012). Automatic stabilizers and economic crisis: US vs. Europe. *Journal of Public Economics* 96: 279–294.

Doole, G.J. (2012). Cost-effective policies for improving water quality by reducing nitrate emissions from diverse dairy farms: an abatement–cost perspective. *Agricultural Water Management* 104: 10–20.

Edwards, K.L. and Clarke, G. (2012). Simobesity: combinatorial optimisation (deterministic) model. In: *Spatial Microsimulation: A Reference Guide for Users* (eds. R. Tanton and K. Edwards), 69–85. The Netherlands: Springer.

Feenberg, D.R. and Coutts, E. (1993). An introduction to the TAXSIM model. *Journal of Policy Analysis and Management* 12 (1): 189–194.

Feldstein, M.S. and Feenberg, D.R. (1983). Alternative tax rules and personal saving incentives: Microeconomic data and behavioral simulations. In: *Behavioral Simulation Methods in Tax Policy Analysis* (ed. M.S. Feldstein), 173–210. Chicago, London: University of Chicago Press.

Felsenstein, D., Axhausen, K., and Waddell, P. (2010). Land use-transportation modeling with UrbanSim: experiences and progress. *Journal of Transport and Land Use* 3 (2): 1–3.

Fernández Salgado, M., Figari, F., Sutherland, H., and Tumino, A. (2014). Welfare compensation for unemployment in the Great Recession. *Review of Income and Wealth* 60: S177–S204.

Figari, F. and Paulus, A. (2015). The distributional effects of taxes and transfers under alternative income concepts: the importance of three 'i's. *Public Finance Review* 43 (3): 347–372.

Figari, F., Immervoll, H., Levy, H., and Sutherland, H. (2011a). Inequalities within couples in Europe: market incomes and the role of taxes and benefits. *Eastern Economic Journal* 37: 344–366.

Figari, F., Paulus, A., and Sutherland, H. (2011b). Measuring the size and impact of public cash support for children in cross-national perspective. *Social Science Computer Review* 29 (1): 85–102.

Figari, F., Salvatori, A., and Sutherland, H. (2011c). Economic downturn and stress testing European welfare systems. In: *Who Loses in the Downturn? Economic Crisis, Employment and Income Distribution*, Vol. 32 of Research in Labor Economics (eds. H. Immervoll, A. Peichl and K. Tatsiramos), 257–286. Emerald Group Publishing Limited.

Figari, F., Matsaganis, M., and Sutherland, H. (2013). Are European social safety nets tight enough? Coverage and adequacy of minimum income schemes in 14 EU countries. *International Journal of Social Welfare* 22: 2013.

Figari, F., Paulus, A., and Sutherland, H. (2015). Microsimulation and policy analysis. In: *Handbook of Income Distribution*, vol. 2 (eds. A.B. Atkinson and F. Bourguignon), 2141–2221. Amsterdam: Elsevier.

Figari, F., Paulus, A., Sutherland, H. et al. (2016). Removing homeownership bias in taxation: the distributional effects of including net imputed rent in taxable income. *Fiscal Studies* 38 (4): 525–557.

Fischer, M., Outwater, M., Cheng, L. et al. (2005). Innovative framework for modeling freight transportation in Los Angeles County, California. *Transportation Research Record: Journal of the Transportation Research Board* 1906: 105–112.

Frick, J.R., Grabka, M.M., Smeeding, T.M., and Tsakloglou, P. (2010). Distributional effects of imputed rents in five European countries. *Journal of Housing Economics* 19 (3): 167–179.

Fujii, S. and Gärling, T. (2003). Application of attitude theory for improved predictive accuracy of stated preference methods in travel demand analysis. *Transportation Research Part A: Policy and Practice* 37 (4): 389–402.

Goldman, N. (1978). Estimating the intrinsic rate of increase of population from the average numbers of younger and older sisters. *Demography* 15 (4): 499–507.

Goodman, L.A., Keyfitz, N., and Pullum, T.W. (1974). Family formation and the frequency of various kinship relationships. *Theoretical Population Biology* 5 (1): 1–27.

Hamilton, K. and Cameron, G. (1994). Simulating the distributional effects of a Canadian carbon tax. *Canadian Public Policy/Analyse de Politiques* 20 (4): 385–399.

Hammel, E.A. and Wachter, K.W. (1996). Evaluating the Slavonian census of 1698 Part II: a microsimulation test and extension of the evidence. *European Journal of Population/Revue européenne de Démographie* 12 (4): 295–326.

Hammel, E.A., McDaniel, C.K., and Wachter, K.W. (1979). Demographic consequences of incest tabus: a microsimulation analysis. *Science* 205 (4410): 972–977.

Hammel, E.A., Mason, C., Wachter, K.W. et al. (1991). Rapid population change and kinship: the effects of unstable demographic changes on Chinese kinship networks, 1750-2250. In: *Consequences of Rapid Population Growth in Developing Countries*, 243–271. New York: Taylor and Francis.

Hanley, N., Colombo, S., Tinch, D. et al. (2006). Estimating the benefits of water quality improvements under the Water Framework Directive: are benefits transferable? *European Review of Agricultural Economics* 33 (3): 391–413.

Harding, A., Vu, Q.N., Tanton, R., and Vidyattama, Y. (2009). Improving work incentives and incomes for parents: the national and geographic impact of liberalising the family tax benefit income test. *Economic Record* 85 (s1): S48–S58.

Herault, N. (2007). Trade liberalisation, poverty and inequality in South Africa: a computable general equilibrium-microsimulation analysis*. *Economic Record* 83 (262): 317–328.

Hérault, N., Kalb, G., and van Zijll de Jong, M. (2009). *Linking a Dynamic CGE Model and a Microsimulation Model: Climate Change Mitigation Policies and Income Distribution in Australia*. Melbourne Institute of Applied Economic and Social Research, University of Melbourne.

Hungerford, T.L. (2010). The redistributive effect of selected federal transfer and tax provisions. *Public Finance Review* 38 (4): 450–472.

Hynes, S. and O'Donoghue, C. (2014). Environmental models. In: *Handbook of Microsimulation Modeling* (ed. C. O'Donoghue), 449–477. Bingley: Emerald.

Hynes, S., Hanley, N., and O'Donoghue, C. (2009a). Alternative treatments of the cost of time in recreational demand models: an application to white-water kayaking in Ireland. *Journal of Environmental Management* 90 (2): 1014–1021.

Hynes, S., Morrissey, K., O'Donoghue, C., and Clarke, G. (2009b). A spatial micro-simulation analysis of methane emissions from Irish agriculture. *Ecological Complexity* 6 (2): 135–146.

Hynes, S., Morrissey, K., and O'Donoghue, C. (2013). Modeling greenhouse gas emissions from agriculture. In: *Spatial Microsimulation for Rural Policy Analysis* (eds. K. Morrissey, C. O'Donoghue, S. Hynes, et al.), 143–157. Berlin Heidelberg: Springer.

Immervoll, H. and O'Donoghue, C. (2004). What difference does a job make? The income consequences of joblessness in Europe. In: *Resisting Marginalisation: Unemployment Experience and Social Policy in the European Union*, Chapter 5 (ed. D. Gallie), 105–137. Oxford: Oxford University Press.

Immervoll, H., Kleven, H.J., Kreiner, C.T., and Saez, E. (2007). Welfare reform in European countries: a microsimulation analysis. *The Economic Journal* 117 (516): 1–44.

Immervoll, H., Kleven, H.J., Kreiner, C.T., and Verdelin, N. (2011). Optimal tax and transfer programs for couples with extensive labor supply responses. *Journal of Public Economics* 95 (11–12): 1485–1500.

Jara, H.X. and Tumino, A. (2013). Tax-benefit systems, income distribution and work incentives in the European Union. *International Journal of Microsimulation* 6 (1): 27–62.

Johnston, R.J. and Rosenberger, R.S. (2010). Methods, trends and controversies in contemporary benefit transfer. *Journal of Economic Surveys* 24 (3): 479–510.

Kask, S.B. and Shogren, J.F. (1994). Benefit transfer protocol for long-term health risk valuation: a case of surface water contamination. *Water Resources Research* 30 (10): 2813–2823.

Kass, G.V. (1980). An exploratory technique for investigating large quantities of categorical data. *Applied Statistics* 29 (2): 119–127.

Keane, M.P. and Moffitt, R. (1998). A structural model of multiple welfare program participation and labor supply. *International Economic Review* 39 (3): 553–589.

King, M.A. (1983). The distribution of gains and losses from changes in the tax treatment of housing. In: *Behavioural Simulation Methods in Tax Policy Analysis* (ed. M. Feldstein), 109–138. Chicago, IL: University of Chicago Press.

Kitamura, R. and Fujii, S. (1998). Two computational process models of activity-travel behavior. In: *Theoretical Foundations of Travel Choice Modeling* (eds. T. Garling, T. Laitila and K. Westin), 251–279. Emerald Group Publishing Limited.

Kongmuang, C., Clarke, G. P., Evans, A. J. and Jin, J. (2006). SimCrime: A spatial microsimulation model for the analysing of crime in Leeds. Working Paper 06/1. School of Geography, University of Leeds, UK.

Labandeira, X. and Labeaga, J. (1999). Combining input-output analysis and micro-simulation to assess the effects of carbon taxation on Spanish households. *Fiscal Studies* 20 (3): 305–320.

Labandeira, X., Labeaga, J.M., and Rodríguez, M. (2007). *Microsimulation in the Analysis of Environmental Tax Reforms. An Application for Spain. Microsimulation as a tool for the evaluation of public policies: methods and applications.* Madrid: Fundación BBVA.

Lal, R. and Follett, R.F. (eds.) (2009). Soil carbon sequestration and the greenhouse effect (No. 57). ASA-CSSA-SSSA.

Ledoux, L. and Turner, R.K. (2002). Valuing ocean and coastal resources: a review of practical examples and issues for further action. *Ocean & Coastal Management* 45 (9): 583–616.

Leontief, W.W. (1951). Input-output economics. *Scientific American* 185 (4): 15–21.

Lesthaeghe, R. (1995). The second demographic transition in Western countries: an interpretation. *Gender and Family Change in Industrialized Countries* (pp. 17–62). Interuniversity Programme in Demography – Working Paper 1991-2. Centrum Sociologie, Vrije Universiteit Brussel, Brussel

Lin, J. (1994). Parity and security: a simulation study of old-age support in rural China. *Population and Development Review* 20 (2): 423–448.

Lin, J. (1995). Changing kinship structure and its implications for old-age support in urban and rural China. *Population Studies* 49 (1): 127–145.

Lymer, S., Brown, L., Yap, M., and Harding, A. (2008). 2001 regional disability estimates for New South Wales, Australia, using spatial microsimulation. *Applied Spatial Analysis and Policy* 1 (2): 99–116.

Lymer, S., Brown, L., Harding, A., and Yap, M. (2009). Predicting the need for aged care services at the small area level: the CAREMOD spatial microsimulation model. *International Journal of Microsimulation* 2 (2): 27–42.

Maestri, V. (2013). Imputed rent and distributional effects of housing-related policies in Estonia, Italy and the United Kingdom. *Baltic Journal of Economics* 13 (2): 35–58.

Mason, C. (2014). Demographic models. In: *Handbook of Microsimulation Modeling* (ed. C. O'Donoghue), 345–365. Bingley: Emerald.

Matsaganis, M. and Flevotomou, M. (2008). A basic income for housing? Simulating a universal housing transfer in the Netherlands and Sweden. *Basic Income Studies* 2 (2): 5–5.

Matsaganis, M. and Leventi, C. (2014). The distributional impact of austerity and the recession in Southern Europe. *South European Society and Politics* 19 (3): 393–412.

McDaniel, C.K. and Hammel, E.A. (1984). A kin-based measure of *r* and an evaluation of its effectiveness. *Demography* 21 (1): 41–51.

McQuinn, K. and Binfield, J. (2002). Estimating the marginal cost to Irish agriculture of reductions in greenhouse gases. Rural Economy Research Centre, working paper. Teagasc, Dublin.

Meyer, M.D. and Miller, E.J. (2001). *Urban Transportation Planning: A Decision-Oriented Approach*. New York: McGraw-Hill College.

Miller, E. and Roorda, M. (2003). Prototype model of household activity-travel scheduling. *Transportation Research Record: Journal of the Transportation Research Board* 1831: 114–121.

Minot, N. and Baulch, B. (2005). Poverty mapping with aggregate census data: what is the loss in precision? *Review of Development Economics* 9 (1): 5–24.

Mitchell, G. (1999). Demand forecasting as a tool for sustainable water resource management. *International Journal of Sustainable Development & World Ecology* 6 (4): 231–241.

Mohanty, I., Tanton, R., Vidyattama, Y. et al. (2013). *Small Area Estimates of Subjective Wellbeing: Spatial Microsimulation on the Australian Unity Wellbeing Index Survey (No. 13/23)*. University of Canberra, National Centre for Social and Economic Modeling.

Murphy, M. (2010). Changes in family and kinship networks consequent on the demographic transitions in England and Wales. *Continuity and Change* 25 (1): 109–136.

Murphy, M. (2011). Long-term effects of the demographic transition on family and kinship networks in Britain. *Population and Development Review* 37 (s1): 55–80.

Noth, M., Borning, A., and Waddell, P. (2003). An extensible, modular architecture for simulating urban development, transportation, and environmental impacts. *Computers, Environment and Urban Systems* 27 (2): 181–203.

O'Donoghue, C. (1997). Carbon dioxide, energy taxes and household income. Economic and Social Research Institute. Working paper N. 90, Dublin.

O'Donoghue, C., Ballas, D., Clarke, G. et al. (eds.) (2012). *Spatial Microsimulation for Rural Policy Analysis*. Springer Science & Business Media.

Paulus, A. and Peichl, A. (2009). Effects of flat tax reforms in Western Europe. *Journal of Policy Modeling* 31 (5): 620–636.

Paulus, A., Sutherland, H., and Tsakloglou, P. (2010). The distributional impact of in-kind public benefits in European countries. *Journal of Policy Analysis & Management* 29 (2): 243–266.

Paulus, A., Figari, F., and Sutherland, H. (2017). The design of fiscal consolidation measures in the European Union: distributional effects and implications for macroeconomic recovery. *Oxford Economic Papers* 69 (3): 632–654.

Procter, K.L., Clarke, G.P., Ransley, J.K., and Cade, J. (2008). Micro-level analysis of childhood obesity, diet, physical activity, residential socioeconomic and social capital variables: where are the obesogenic environments in Leeds? *Area* 40 (3): 323–340.

Recker, W.W. and Golob, T.F. (1979). A non-compensatory model of transportation behavior based on sequential consideration of attributes. *Transportation Research Part B: Methodological* 13 (4): 269–280.

Robin, T. (2011). New challenges in disaggregate behavioral modeling. PhD thesis. Ecole Polytechnique Federale de Lausanne, Lausanne.

Robinson, D., Haldi, F., Kämpf, J. et al. (2009). CitySim: comprehensive micro-simulation of resource flows for sustainable urban planning. Eleventh International IBPSA Conference, 1083–1090.

Roorda, M.J., Miller, E.J., and Habib, K.M. (2008). Validation of TASHA: a 24-h activity scheduling microsimulation model. *Transportation Research Part A: Policy and Practice* 42 (2): 360–375.

Rosenberger, R.S. and Loomis, J.B. (2001). Benefit Transfer of Outdoor Recreation Use Values: A Technical Document Supporting the Forest Service Strategic Plan (2000 Revision). *General Technical Report, N. RMRS-GTR-72, Rocky Mountain Research Station, USDA Forest Service.*

Ruggles, S. (1987). *Prolonged Connections: the Rise of the Extended Family in Nineteenth-Century England and America*. Madison, WI: University of Wisconsin Press.

Sahaleh, S., Bierlaire, M., Farooq, B. et al. (2012). Scenario analysis of pedestrian flow in public spaces. *In 12th Swiss Transport Research Conference* (No. EPFL-CONF-181239).

Salanauskaite, L. and Verbist, G. (2013). Is the neighbour's grass greener? Comparing family support in Lithuania and four other New Member States. *Journal of European Social Policy* 23 (3): 315–331.

Sander, B., Nizam, A., Garrison, L.P. et al. (2009). Economic evaluation of influenza pandemic mitigation strategies in the United States using a stochastic microsimulation transmission model. *Value in Health* 12 (2): 226–233.

Ševčíková, H., Raftery, A.E., and Waddell, P.A. (2007). Assessing uncertainty in urban simulations using Bayesian melding. *Transportation Research Part B: Methodological* 41 (6): 652–669.

Simon, H.A. (1957). *Models of Man; Social and Rational*. New York: Wiley.

Smith, J.E. (1991). *Aging Together, Aging Alone. Life Span Extension: Consequences and Open Questions*, 81–92. New York: Springer Publishing Company.

Smith, V.E. and Strauss, J. (1986). Simulating the rural economy in a subsistence environment: Sierra Leone. In: *Agricultural Household Models: Extensions, Applications, and Policy* (eds. I. Singh, L. Squire and J. Strauss), 206–232. Baltimore and London: The Johns Hopkins University Press.

Smith, D.M., Pearce, J.R., and Harland, K. (2011). Can a deterministic spatial microsimulation model provide reliable small-area estimates of health behaviours? An example of smoking prevalence in New Zealand. *Health & Place* 17 (2): 618–624.

van Soest, A. (1995). Structural models of family labor supply: a discrete choice approach. *The Journal of Human Resources* 30 (1): 63–88.

Sutherland, H. and Figari, F. (2013). EUROMOD: the European Union tax-benefit microsimulation model. *International Journal of Microsimulation* 6 (1): 4–26.

Symons, E., Proops, J., and Gay, P. (1994). Carbon taxes, consumer demand and carbon dioxide emissions: a simulation analysis for the UK. *Fiscal Studies* 15 (2): 19–43.

Tanton, R. (2014). A review of spatial microsimulation methods. *International Journal of Microsimulation* 7 (1): 4–25.

Tanton, R., Harding, A., and Mcnamara, J. (2010). Urban and rural estimates of poverty: recent advances in spatial microsimulation in Australia. *Geographical Research* 48 (1): 52–64.

Tanton, R., Vidyattama, Y., Nepal, B., and McNamara, J. (2011). Small area estimation using a reweighting algorithm. *Journal of the Royal Statistical Society: Series A (Statistics in Society)* 174 (4): 931–951.

Tanton, R., Harding, A., and McNamara, J. (2013). Spatial microsimulation using a generalised regression model. In: *Spatial Microsimulation: A Reference Guide for Users* (eds. R. Tanton and K. Edwards), 87–103. Dordrecht: Springer.

Tomintz, M.N., Clarke, G.P., and Rigby, J.E. (2008). The geography of smoking in Leeds: estimating individual smoking rates and the implications for the location of stop smoking services. *Area* 40 (3): 341–353.

Tomintz, M.N., Clarke, G.P., and Rigby, J.E. (2009). Planning the location of stop smoking services at the local level: a geographic analysis. *Journal of Smoking Cessation* 4 (2): 61–73.

Tomintz, M.N., Clarke, G.P., Rigby, J.E., and Green, J.M. (2013). Optimising the location of antenatal classes. *Midwifery* 29 (1): 33–43.

Tversky, A. (1972). Elimination by aspects: a theory of choice. *Psychological Review* 79 (4): 281–299.

Vasic, J. and Ruskin, H.J. (2011). A discrete flow simulation model for urban road networks, with application to combined car and single-file bicycle traffic. In: *Computational Science and Its Applications-ICCSA 2011* (eds. B. Murgante, O. Gervasi, A. Iglesias, et al.), 602–614. Berlin Heidelberg: Springer.

Verbist, G. (2007). The distribution effect of taxes on pensions and unemployment benefits in the EU-15. In: *Microsimulation In Action: Policy Analysis in Europe using EUROMOD*, Vol. 25 of Research In Labor Economics (ed. O. Bargain), 73–99. Elsevier.

Verbist, G. and Figari, F. (2014). The redistributive effect and progressivity of taxes revisited: an international comparison across the European Union. *FinanzArchiv/ Public Finance Analysis* 70 (3): 405–429.

Vidyattama, Y. and Tanton, R. (2010). Projecting small area statistics with Australian spatial microsimulation model (SpatialMSM). *Australasian Journal of Regional Studies* 16 (1): 99.

Vidyattama, Y. and Tanton, R. (2013). Projections using a static spatial microsimulation model. In: *Spatial Microsimulation: A Reference Guide for Users* (eds. R. Tanton and K. Edwards), 145–160. The Netherlands: Springer.

Vidyattama, Y., Cassells, R., Harding, A., and Mcnamara, J. (2013). Rich or poor in retirement? A small area analysis of Australian private superannuation savings in 2006 using spatial microsimulation. *Regional Studies* 47 (5): 722–739.

Vu, Q.N. and Tanton, R. (2010). The distributional and regional impact of the Australian Government's Household Stimulus Package. *Australasian Journal of Regional Studies* 16 (1): 127.

Wachter, K.W. (1980). The sisters' riddle and the importance of variance when guessing demographic rates from kin counts. *Demography* 17 (1): 103–114.

Wachter, K.W. (1997). Kinship resources for the elderly. *Philosophical Transactions of the Royal Society of London B: Biological Sciences* 352 (1363): 1811–1817.

Wachter, K.W., Knodel, J.E., and VanLandingham, M. (2002). AIDS and the elderly of Thailand: projecting familial impacts. *Demography* 39 (1): 25–41.

Waduda, Z., Noland, R.B., and Graham, D.J. (2008). Equity analysis of personal tractable carbon permits for the road transport sector. *Environmental Science and Policy* 11 (6): 533–544.

Williams, H.C.W.L. and Ortúzar, J.D.D. (1982). Behavioural theories of dispersion and the mis-specification of travel demand models. *Transportation Research Part B: Methodological* 16 (3): 167–219.

Williamson, P. (2001). An applied microsimulation model: exploring alternative domestic water consumption scenarios. In: *Regional Science in Business*, 243–268. Berlin Heidelberg: Springer.

Williamson, P., Clarke, G.P., and McDonald, A.T. (1996). Estimating small-area demands for water with the use of microsimulation. In: *Microsimulation for Urban and Regional Policy Analysis*, European Research in Regional Science 6 (ed. G.P. Clarke), 117–148. London: Pion.

Williamson, P., Mitchell, G., and McDonald, A.T. (2002). Domestic water demand forecasting: a static microsimulation approach. *Water and Environment Journal* 16 (4): 243–248.

Yusuf, A.A. (2008). The Distributional Impact of Environmental Policy: The Case of Carbon Tax and Energy Pricing Reform in Indonesia. *Research report (2008-RR1)*. Singapore: Environment and Economy Program for Southeast Asia.

Zagheni, E. (2011). The impact of the HIV/AIDS epidemic on orphanhood probabilities and kinship structure in Zimbabwe. *Population and Development Review* 37 (4): 761–783.

Zhang, S., Ren, G., and Yang, R. (2013). Simulation model of speed–density characteristics for mixed bicycle flow – comparison between cellular automata model and gas dynamics model. *Physica A: Statistical Mechanics and its Applications* 392 (20): 5110–5118.

Zhao, Z. (1998). *Demographic Conditions, Microsimulation, and Family Support for the Elderly: Past, Present and Future in China. The Locus of Care: Families, Communities, Institutions, and the Provision of Welfare Since Antiquity*, 259–279. London: Routledge.

Harding, A. (1993). *Lifetime Income Distribution and Redistribution: Applications of a Microsimulation Model. Contributions to Economic Analysis*, vol. 221. Amsterdam: North Holland.

Rozan, A. (2004). Benefit transfer: a comparison of WTP for air quality between France and Germany. *Environmental and Resource Economics* 29: 295–306.

9

Applications of Microsimulation Models to the Social Determinants of Health and Public Health

A Systematic Review of the Literature

Daniel Kim

Bouvé College of Health Sciences, Northeastern University, Boston, MA, USA
School of Public Policy and Urban Affairs, Northeastern University, Boston, MA, USA

9.1 Overview

While the previous chapter reviewed recent and important approaches to and applications of microsimulation in the social sciences, this chapter systematically reviews the application of microsimulation models to the social determinants of health. Through such a review, I aim to identify patterns and gaps in the literature on the social determinants of health and thereby to advance research in these areas. Broadly, this systematic review should help to promote our understanding of the ways in which social determinants may shape health and well-being, and serve to inform the development of more effective interventions and policies to improve population health and reduce health inequalities across the life course.

This systematic review encompasses the empirical literature on each of the contextual and individual-level social determinants of health. To my knowledge, it is the first comprehensive review of empirical applications of microsimulation models to estimating the impacts of the social determinants of health. Using the PubMed search engine, Web of Science database, PsycINFO database, EMBASE database, Scopus database, and Google Scholar from 1966 to 30 April 2018, I systematically reviewed the current evidence on the empirical applications of microsimulation models as they relate to social determinants of population health. The following combinations of keywords/subject headings were applied to identify original articles of macroeconomic and macrosocial social determinants, area-level contextual social determinants, and individual-level social determinants: (microsimulation AND (health OR disease) AND ((social determinants) OR (income inequality) OR (social policy) OR tax OR (neighborhood deprivation) OR (neighborhood socioeconomic status) OR (socioeconomic status) OR race OR (residential segregation) OR (social capital))).

For the purpose of this systematic review, I focus on nonmedical social and economic determinants of health and disease. Because as mentioned in Chapter 1, health care factors are not considered major determinants of population health, I do not review health care as a social determinant. Recent national and international commissioned reports on the social determinants of health, including from the WHO Commission on the Social Determinants of Health (2008) and the Robert Wood Johnson Foundation Commission to Build a Healthier America (2009), have placed primary emphasis on nonmedical societal determinants that span a wide range of health outcomes. An additional criterion for inclusion in this review was publication in the English language. Based on abstracts returned from this search, I reviewed relevant papers and searched their references for additional papers.

In the second part of this review, I employed the same databases to identify key articles in the following areas of empirical applications of microsimulation models to medicine and public health: health care policy (e.g. simulation of health care reform policy proposals), disease microsimulation (e.g. effects of screening/disease on labor force participation, economic costs, and wealth), and health behavior-related policy (e.g. simulation of federal policies on after-school physical activity and soft drink taxation).

Figure 9.1 shows the number of documents published in the Web of Science database using the combined keywords "microsimulation" AND ("health" or

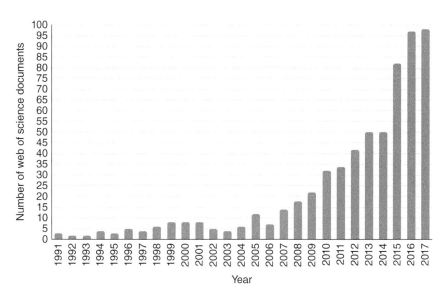

Figure 9.1 Published documents in Web of Science using combined keywords "microsimulation" and ("health" OR "disease"), 1991–2017.

"disease") over time. As seen in this figure, the first document/article appeared in 1991. Since then, there has been a steady rise in the number of items published, with a steeper rise since the mid-2000s.

9.2 Direct Empirical Applications to the Study of the Social Determinants of Health

Based on the above mentioned search engines and databases, I identified a total of 11 published articles or reports (out of 101 documents retrieved through the Web of Science database) that contained direct empirical applications to the study of the social determinants of health. I briefly describe each of these studies below.

Edwards and Clarke (2009) and Procter et al. (2008) used the spatial microsimulation model SimObesity to model childhood obesogenic environmental and behavioral variables at the small area level and to identify small area-level patterns of obesogenic covariates in Leeds, United Kingdom. These variables included factors related to families (e.g. socioeconomic group, expenditures on food, and TV ownership), schools (school meal consumption, dichotomized into whether purchased school meals or not), and neighborhoods (residential urbanization, deprivation, access to local amenities, social capital, and perceived local safety). Individual-level data from the Health Survey for England 2002 and from the Expenditure and Food Survey 2005 were combined with data from the 2001 Census using a reweighting deterministic algorithm, thereby creating a synthetic population of individuals "living" in each small area in Leeds. A key advantage of spatial microsimulation models is their ability to estimate geographical distributions of variables previously unknown, such as the distribution of obese children across households in a city (Procter et al. 2008). Local potential issues can then be highlighted, rather than being obscured if we were to rely on population averages for the larger region. Procter et al. (2008) used spatially-weighted regression to investigate the relationships between different obesogenic environments and childhood obesity, and found that social capital and poverty were both strongly associated with childhood obesity, after taking into account other environmental and individual factors. On average, perceived access to supermarkets and leisure facilities and perceived quality of public transport services were all significantly associated with obesity. However, mapping the results enabled the visualization of spatial variations—that is, being able to see areas where predictors reduced the risks of childhood obesity, and identify other areas (i.e. hot spots) where the relationships appeared to be obesogenic.

Likewise, Koh et al. (2015) employed spatial microsimulation to obtain local estimates of obesity prevalence because national health surveys such as the Centers for Disease Control and Prevention (CDC) Behavioral Risk Factor

Surveillance System (BRFSS) surveys are not designed to produce direct estimates at the local levels due to small population samples. They implemented a spatial microsimulation model to replicate the demographic characteristics of BRFSS respondents to census tract populations in metropolitan Detroit. At the census tract level, obesity prevalence was strongly correlated ($r = 0.54$) with the prevalence of low-income families, defined as a poverty rate of 20% or higher or a median family income less than 80% of the median family income for the metropolitan area. This study provides a useful new methodological approach to assess local areas in need of future obesity interventions.

Ballas et al. (2006) used a dynamic spatial microsimulation model of Britain from the censuses of 1971, 1981, and 1991 and the British Household Panel Survey to simulate urban and regional populations in Britain. In a 30-year simulation that estimated variables such as household income at the small area level, they observed that areas with higher average income levels were less likely to report health problems.

Laditka et al. (2007) applied discrete-time Markov chains and microsimulation modeling to estimate and compare life expectancy and the expected number of years with physical impairment among impaired individuals at baseline and followed for 20 years, according to rural vs. urban residence, gender, race, and education. Rural residents were found to live longer than urban residents, and to live more years with physical impairment and with a larger proportion of remaining life impaired. Stratifying by urban residence, gender, race, and education revealed longer life expectancies in women, in Whites (vs. Blacks), and in those with 12 or more years of education.

In an earlier study that also used Markov chain and microsimulation models, Wolf et al. (2002) explored the distribution of total, unimpaired, and impaired life for multiple groups of older women as defined by race, education, and marital history. Among all groups studied, never-married, more-educated White women lived the longest, healthiest lives. Ever-married non-White women with lower education had the shortest average life expectancy, and they were found to experience the most disability. These results highlight the large heterogeneity of disability processes and life expectancy for older women.

Employing a dynamic microsimulation model, Lay-Yee et al. (2015) simulated health care and health-related outcomes in a New Zealand cohort of children born in 1977. They modeled structural social determinants including parental race/ethnicity and education and parental income (employment and welfare dependence) as predictors of health service use (family doctor visits) and educational and social outcomes (reading ability and conduct disorder). Based on this microsimulation, they determined that modifying structural determinants were relatively more important than intermediary ones as potential policy levers, that there was a social gradient, and that the most disadvantaged groups benefited the most with a corresponding reduction in disparities between the worst off and the best off.

Coupling longitudinal microdata from the National Population Health Survey (Statistics Canada) with microsimulation, Wolfson and Rowe (2014) investigated the relative importance of selected determinants of population health. Health-adjusted life expectancy (HALE), which is an aggregation of individuals' adjusted-health life lengths, was the outcome. They used longitudinal microsimulation to synthesize a nationally-representative longitudinal population sample of Canadians, and then constructed a series of counterfactual populations. Through comparisons between and among counterfactuals and the base case, they then estimated the quantitative importance of various factors in determining HALE. Wolfson and Rowe (2014) examined four specific risk factors: obesity, smoking, education, and sense of coherence. Of these factors, obesity appeared to have the smallest impacts on HALE: moving from the 5th to the 95th percentiles of body mass index (BMI) was expected to increase HALE by 1.5 and 2.5 years for men and women, respectively. Eliminating smoking was predicted to increase HALE by five and four years, whereas moving from the lowest to the highest levels of education would have comparable effects of five years for both men and women. Somewhat surprisingly, moving from the 5th to the 95th percentiles of the psychosocial factor of sense of coherence was expected to have the largest impact on HALE, with estimated increases of 5.5–6 years. These results reinforce the relative importance of education as well as psychosocial factors as determinants of health and the comparatively smaller impacts of more proximal intermediary risk factors such as obesity and smoking.

The National Centre for Social and Economic Modeling (NATSEM) in Australia used MSM to estimate the potential economic cost savings and population health benefits that would occur if the WHO's recommendations on the social determinants of health were to be adopted in Australia (National Centre for Social and Economic Modeling, 2012). The costs of government inaction were estimated based on the loss of potential social and economic gains that otherwise would hypothetically have accrued to socioeconomically disadvantaged individuals if they had the same health profile of more socioeconomically advantaged Australians. Using microsimulation modeling, disadvantaged individuals were counterfactually shifted from poor to good health to match the average health profile of the most advantaged group. Among other findings in this published report, they projected that 500 000 Australians could avoid suffering a chronic illness; 170 000 extra Australians could enter the workforce, generating $8 billion in extra earnings; annual savings of $4 billion in welfare support payments could be made; and that 60 000 fewer people would need to be admitted to hospital annually, resulting in an overall savings of $2.3 billion in hospital expenditures. The data to assess potential savings to the health system were derived from three of NATSEM's health microsimulation models: HospMod (a static microsimulation model of utilization and costs of hospitals in Australia; MediSim (a static microsimulation model of the utilization and costs of the Australian Pharmaceutical Benefits Scheme; and the APPSIM health module (a module within the dynamic microsimulation model APPSIM that simulates lifestyle risk factors, self-reported health status, and health service utilization and costs in Australia) (National Centre for Social and Economic Modeling, 2012). These data were supplemented with administrative data from Medicare Australia. Notably, this microsimulation analysis assumed that all of the health differences between socioeconomically advantaged and disadvantaged groups were attributable to social determinants of health, although they did not examine the impacts according to specific social determinants of health.

In an interrupted time-series analysis, Muennig et al. (2016) explored the impacts of state-level incremental supplements to the Earned Income Tax Credit (EITC) program on health-related quality of life using data from the 1993 to 2010 BRFSS surveys and state-level average life expectancy. The cost-effectiveness of state EITC supplements was estimated using a Markov microsimulation model. This model accounted for annual losses associated with cash transfers from higher to lower income groups (i.e. deadweight loss) and incremental changes in quality-adjusted life expectancy associated with EITC supplementation. Overall, supplemental EITC programs were predicted to increase health-related quality of life and longevity among the poor and appeared to be highly cost-effective—with the program costing roughly $7786 per quality-adjusted life-year gained for the average recipient.

In a recent tax microsimulation analysis, Kim (2018) projected the impacts on mortality of modifying federal income tax structures based on proposals by two recent US presidential candidates: Donald Trump and Senator Bernie Sanders. He performed a microsimulation analysis using the latest U.S. Internal Revenue Service public-use tax file with state identifiers (2008 tax year), containing nationally representative data from 139 651 tax returns and TAXSIM, a static tax microsimulation model. This microsimulation analysis considered five tax plan scenarios: (i) actual 2008 tax structures; proposals in 2016 by then-candidates (ii) Trump and (iii) Sanders; (iv) a modified Sanders plan with higher top tax rates (75%); and (v) a modified Sanders plan with higher top rates plus revenue redistribution to lower income households (<$40 000/year). Combining projected changes in income inequality with vital statistics data and past estimates of linkages between income inequality, income, and mortality, he estimated there would be 29 689 (95% CI: 10 865–48 920) more deaths/year and 31 302 (95% CI: 11 455–51 577) fewer deaths/year from all causes under the Trump and Sanders plans, respectively. Under the modified Sanders plan including higher top rates, he projected 68 919 (95% CI: 25 221–113 561) fewer deaths/year. Under the modified Sanders plan with redistribution, he estimated 333 504 (95% CI:

192 897–473 787) fewer deaths/year. Overall, this study concluded that policies that both raise federal income tax rates and redistribute tax revenue could confer large reductions in the total number of annual deaths among Americans, and that policymakers should consider joint federal tax and redistributive policies as levers to reduce the burden of mortality in the United States (Kim 2018).

9.3 Other Empirical Applications of Microsimulation Models to Medicine and Public Health

Health Care Policy Models

Microsimulation models have further been used in health services research to model health care reform policy proposals. Health care reform takes the form of policies including expansions in coverage to uninsured populations; possible public insurance coverage of prescription drugs and/or long-term care; varying levels of patient copayments; and changes in the type and level of payment to health care providers (e.g. salary, fee-for-service, and capitation) (Glied and Tilipman 2010). Modeled outcomes of interest have included changes in the population percentage of health care insurance coverage (private and public), health care utilization, health care provider participation, quality and outcomes of care (Cordova et al. 2013), and costs. The latter includes direct health care expenditures (expressed as total costs or costs per newly insured person, which can be used in cost-effectiveness analyses), as well as costs as a result of changes in the tax code, and costs associated with provider subsidies for uncompensated costs. Furthermore, costs are incurred by nongovernmental payers, including individuals and employers (Glied and Tilipman 2010). Finally, the consequences of reform have been estimated for population subgroups such as those defined by demographic characteristics (e.g. age, sex, and race/ethnicity), socioeconomic status, and geography of residence (e.g. state, county, and metropolitan statistical area).

As an example, the Gruber Microsimulation Model (GMSIM) has been used to estimate the effects of comprehensive health care reform in the state of Massachusetts in 2008 and subsequently in the entire United States under the Affordable Care Act in 2010. Microsimulation analyses prior to both implementations suggested that among low-income families, there was adequate "room" in their budgets to pay health insurance premiums and to take up employer-sponsored insurance when offered to them at a premium cost, i.e. very low-income families could afford to pay toward their health insurance coverage (Gruber and Seif 2009).

Disease Microsimulation Models

Disease microsimulation models have been widely used to model the effects of disease on labor force participation, direct costs, and wealth. For example, the Health&WealthMOD static microsimulation model (Schofield et al. 2009) was Australia's first microsimulation model of health and disability. This model has been employed to project the impacts that illnesses would have on labor force participation, personal income, and government revenues and expenditures in Australian workers aged 45–64 years. The base population of Health&WealthMOD consists of participants aged 45–65 years from the Survey of Disability, Aging and Carers conducted by the Australian Bureau of Statistics in 2003. Information gathered for each individual includes demographic factors (e.g. age, sex, family type, state of residence, and ethnic background), socioeconomic factors (level of education, income, and benefits received), labor force (labor force participation, employment restrictions, and retirement), and health and disability characteristics (e.g. chronic conditions, health status, and type of disability). Information on income and wealth comes from STINMOD—a separate microsimulation model of income tax and government support payments—and is matched to persons with similar characteristics in Health&WealthMOD to impute economic information onto the base data (Schofield et al. 2009). Sex, income unit type, type of government pension/support, income quintile, age group, labor force status, weekly hours worked, highest educational attainment, and home ownership are employed as matching variables. The microdata are then aged to represent the entire Australian population aged 45–64 years in 2009. In addition, for each individual in Health&WealthMOD, the Survey of Disability, Aging and Carers provides in-depth self-reported data on sociodemographic characteristics, labor force participation, and health and disability status including chronic conditions according to International Classification of Diseases, 10th Revision (ICD-10) codes (Schofield et al. 2009).

The POpulation HEalth Model (POHEM) is a dynamic microsimulation model developed by Statistics Canada in the 1990s. POHEM enables the simulation of life course dynamics and health outcomes of the Canadian population by incorporating multivariate data collected from a variety of sources and projecting counterfactual population distributions of health outcomes based on a population intervention (Hennessy et al. 2015). POHEM models have been developed for diseases and conditions including cardiovascular disease, major cancers (screening, treatment, and costs), osteoarthritis, physical activity, and neurological conditions.

As a dynamic microsimulation model, POHEM simulates determinants, risk factors, and disease states to project health outcomes including disease incidence, prevalence, life expectancy, health-related quality of life, and health care costs (Hennessy et al. 2015). POHEM simulates competing discrete events such as changes in disease states in continuous time. The simulated life trajectory of each individual is influenced by exposure to simulated events such as changes in lifestyle risk factors and onset of disease.

Most of the current POHEM models are initialized based on the 2001 Canadian Community Health Survey and weighted to represent the entire Canadian population over the age of 20 years (Hennessy et al. 2015). Variables include sociodemographic and socioeconomic characteristics (e.g. age, sex, ethnicity, education, and income), risk factors (e.g. BMI, diabetes, smoking, and hypertension), and health status variables (e.g. history of selected diseases). These variables provide starting values for individuals' attributes which are updated and transitioned (Hennessy et al. 2015). After the start-up population is established, individuals' disease states, risk factors, and health determinants are dynamically modeled.

After dynamic updates and risk transitions are applied, estimates of the health outcomes of interest are validated. The POHEM model is validated externally such as by comparing POHEM projections against estimates from hospital data (Canadian Institute for Health Information Discharge Abstract Database) and cancer incidence rates from the Canadian Cancer Registry, and then calibrated as needed in order that simulated estimates more closely approximate observed estimates (Hennessy et al. 2015). Once the model has been validated, calibrated, and a "base-case" projection has been made, counterfactual analysis can then be performed. Counterfactual scenarios include implementing hypothetical interventions such as reducing smoking prevalence or BMI and modeling future impacts on disease incidence.

Michaud et al. (2011) employed an extension of the Future Elderly Model (FEM) to make projections of health and health care costs for all Americans aged 50+ years based on data from the 1992 to 2004 biennial waves of the Health and Retirement Study. Markov modeling was used to transition across health and economic states as a function of risk and demographic factors. The model simulated a range of health and economic outcomes for individuals including life expectancy, healthy life expectancy, and medical expenditures by the federal government. Importantly, this model was also used to simulate the counterfactual case of American health status being at the same levels at baseline as European health status, simulate transitions until everyone died, and then compare this to the status quo scenario of American health. Based on this simulation, Michaud et al. (2011) were able to explain nearly all (92%) of the difference in life expectancy between the United States and Europe. Taking into account the estimated medical care costs and the cost of drugs (using data from the Medical Expenditure Panel Survey and the Medicare Current Beneficiary Survey), tax revenues, Supplemental Security Income (SSI), and medical expenditures on Medicare, Medicaid, for the age 50+ years population, old age pension benefits would increase considerably ($6593 per capita). However, this was more than offset by a larger decrease in

Medicare, Medicaid, and Disability insurance benefit payments: The total lifetime health care expenditures were projected to decrease by a striking $17 791 per capita, or an 8.5% reduction. On average, lifetime payments for Medicare would be reduced by $4717 per capita and for Medicaid by $3687 per capita. Overall, they estimated that this scenario would lead to a net increase in per capita revenue of $4902 for the government (Michaud et al. 2011).

Health Behavior-Related Policy

Several studies have simulated the impacts of policies directed at specific lifestyle behaviors to improve population health. For example, Kristensen et al. (2014) estimated microsimulation models to simulate the effects of federal policies on afterschool physical activity, soft drink taxes, and bans on TV advertising for children. The policies (and corresponding estimated effect sizes) were identified through a systematic review process in which the literature on 26 recommended policies for preventing childhood obesity were examined and then narrowed down to three policies based on criteria of effectiveness, potential population reach, feasibility, acceptability, precision of information, and potential impact on childhood obesity. The three policies were as follows: (i) strengthening and expanding federally funded afterschool programs to promote physical activity; (ii) enacting a $0.01/ounce excise tax on sugar-sweetened beverages (SSB); and (iii) banning fast-food TV advertising targeting children aged 12 years and younger. Afterschool physical activity programs were projected to reduce obesity the most among children aged 6–12 years (1.8 percentage points) and the advertising ban to reduce obesity the least (0.9 percentage points). The microsimulation model, developed in TreeAge (TreeAge Software, Inc.), first drew randomly from a representative sample of simulated school-aged children (6–12 years) and adolescents (13–18 years) based on 2010 U.S. Census data. Over a 20-year period, it then simulated annual changes in physical activity, diet, and BMI using multivariate models based on continuous National Health and Nutrition Examination Survey (NHANES) data (2001–2010). Of the three policies that were explored, the SSB excise tax was predicted to reduce obesity the most among adolescents aged 13–18 years (2.4 percentage points). All three policies were projected to reduce obesity to a greater degree among Blacks and Hispanics than among Whites.

Gortmaker et al. (2015) used microsimulation modeling to estimate the cost-effectiveness of nationally implementing seven obesity prevention interventions high on the child obesity policy agenda: an SSB excise tax; eliminating the tax subsidy for advertising unhealthy foods to children; restaurant menu calorie labeling; nutrition standards for school meals; nutrition standards for all other food and beverages sold in schools; improved early care and education; and increased access to adolescent bariatric surgery. Based on a stochastic, discrete-time, individual-level microsimulation model, the simulation calculated the costs and effectiveness of the interventions through their impacts on BMI, obesity prevalence, and obesity-related health care costs between 2015 and 2025. Data were drawn from the U.S. Census as well as multiple surveys including the BRFSS, NHANESs, the National Survey of Children's Health, and the National Longitudinal Survey of Youth. Implementing these three interventions was projected to prevent anywhere between 129 000 and 576 000 cases of childhood obesity in 2025 (Gortmaker et al. 2015). By contrast, adolescent bariatric surgery had no sizeable impact on obesity prevalence. In addition, three of the interventions—an SSB excise tax, eliminating the tax deduction, and nutrition standards for school meals—were estimated to reduce health care costs more than the cost to implement them. Hence, these results provide empirical evidence to support the importance of primary prevention for policymakers aiming to reduce childhood obesity (Gortmaker et al. 2015).

Tam et al. (2018) proposed to simulate the impacts of tobacco control policies on smoking prevalence and mortality and life-years in the United States using an extension of the Smoking History Generator (SHG), a microsimulation model that draws on data from the National Health Interview Surveys. The SHG simulates life trajectories for individuals including smoking initiation, cessation, and mortality. Four types of tobacco control policies are considered at the national and state levels: smoke-free air laws, cigarette taxes, tobacco control program expenditures, and raising the minimum age of legal access to tobacco (Tam et al. 2018). Smoking prevalence, the number of population deaths avoided, and life-years gained are calculated for each policy scenario at the national and state levels. The researchers are also developing a web-based interface that allows users to explore model outcomes for each policy, either for each state or across the United States, including modifying the policy inputs across a range of values.

Other research has used microsimulation models to explore the impacts of salt reduction policies on primary prevention of cardiovascular disease and gastric cancer in England (Kypridemos et al. 2017) and on CVD deaths, incidence, and quality-adjusted life-years (QALYs) in the United States (Pearson-Stuttard et al. 2018); of increases in meat price in the US adult population on BMI, mortality, and quality of life (Pitt and Bendavid 2017); and of interventions aimed at reducing intake of added sugars on population disease prevalence (liver cirrhosis, obesity, diabetes, and heart disease; Vreman et al. 2017).

Finally, additional studies have estimated the impacts of taxing foods such as SSB in the United States (Basu et al. 2013a); tobacco taxation in India (Basu et al. 2013b) that contribute to obesity and chronic diseases such as diabetes and heart disease; and subsidizing fruit and vegetable purchases nationwide in the United States among Supplemental Nutrition Assistance Program (SNAP) participants on chronic disease morbidity, mortality, and costs over long time horizons (Choi et al. 2017).

9.4   Chapter Summary

This chapter has reviewed a variety of empirical studies of microsimulation in the field of public health, ranging from studies that projected impacts of directly modifying social determinants of health to impacts of health care policies, of disease on labor force participation, direct costs, and wealth, and of health behavior-related policies.

If we take stock and refer back to the conceptual diagram of the social determinants of health depicted in Figure 1.1 in Chapter 1, social determinants of health are considered fundamental social conditions that shape more proximal intermediary determinants of health such as health behaviors. The review in the present chapter finds that there are few microsimulation studies to date that have directly examined the social determinants of health, and suggests that they are currently far outnumbered by studies on intermediary determinants of health and health care combined, as well as disease microsimulation studies. This imbalance in empirical work runs counter to the relative importance that the social determinants of health have in shaping the health of societies. In addition, less than a handful of microsimulation studies have been conducted on the social determinants of health in the United States.

Nonetheless, the microsimulation studies of the social determinants of health conducted to date share some common threads. For example, a couple of studies have compared and contrasted the impacts of social determinants of health to intermediary determinants (Wolfson and Rowe 2014; Lay-Yee et al. 2015). Meanwhile, other studies have focused on the impacts of economic policies such as the EITC and federal taxation (Muennig et al. 2016; Kim 2018). Studies have also taken the critical step of translating these impacts into human costs (e.g. number of lives that would be saved; National Centre for Social and Economic Modeling 2012; Kim 2018) and economic costs (e.g. cost-effectiveness; Muennig et al. 2016) for "what-if" scenarios of intervening on the social determinants of health.

Intermediary determinant studies have focused on interventions and policies including taxation that could help prevent obesity in childhood, smoking, and shape lifestyle risk factors for adult chronic conditions such as diabetes, heart disease, and obesity—including the consumption of salt, meat, and fruits and vegetables. These types of studies can tell us what may work and may not work if we were to intervene on more proximal factors and play an important role along with studies on the social determinants of health. Likewise, microsimulation studies of health care policies can simulate the possible impacts of future policy changes in the health care system that thereby can help to improve patient outcomes and curb the current trajectory of skyrocketing health care system costs. Such studies on intermediary determinants of health including health behaviors and health care policies are still meaningful. But the critical issue is the current apparent shortfall of SDOH microsimulation studies.

This review also reveals some other unexplored empirical gaps in the literature. Of social determinants of health that have been examined so far, several social determinants have yet to be considered through MSM. These social determinants include racial/economic segregation, social spending, and social policies under consideration by some policymakers such as minimum wage and paid family leave policies. Only one study, conducted in Australia, has explored the impacts of adopting the WHO recommendations on the social determinants of health, although as noted earlier it did not examine the impacts of specific determinants. Conducting similar studies in other western industrialized nations including the United States would help fill an evidence void. Issues of bias and limitations of causal inference are also an inherent challenge—notably, MSM simulations have largely relied on data based on observational study designs for which such causal inference challenges apply. Still, as highlighted in Chapter 1, innovative approaches have been implemented in observational studies to address such biases, such as inverse probability weighting and marginal structural models (Thoemmes and Ong 2016) and fixed effects and instrumental variable analysis (Kim 2016). Just as meta-analyses are only as good as the quality of the studies that are included in them ("garbage in = garbage out"; Egger et al. 2001), the quality of microsimulation studies is dependent on the quality of the epidemiological studies that contribute to them. Hence, where possible, the quality of underlying epidemiological studies, particularly as it relates to potential biases, should be measured and presented (e.g. as required by a reporting statement such as STROBE) in published MSM studies. Finally, economic evaluations such as cost-benefit and cost-effectiveness analyses have been sparsely conducted in MSM studies to date. Because of their importance as a relevant metric to policymakers who typically facing tight fiscal constraints, more economic evaluations should be integrated into future MSM research.

In future microsimulation research, one promising avenue is to integrate aspects of spatial microsimulation, disease microsimulation, health care policy, and/or social policy microsimulation into the same analyses. For example, so far disease microsimulation models have not considered the impacts of contextual social determinants of health including social and economic policies. Yet disease microsimulation models that make projections over long time horizons offer powerful tools for studying the longitudinal impacts of contextual social determinants on disease incidence and mortality. Employing aspects of health care policy simulation models might also help us to better understand the impacts on the health care system and on population health. Extending the approach combining spatial microsimulation and tax–benefit simulation mentioned in Chapter 7 (Tanton et al. 2009) to include health estimates, one could project small area population health changes as a result of tax–benefit policy changes. Relatedly, Schofield et al. (2018) have referred to MSM applications built for one purpose and then through linkages to other data applied for another purpose as "cross-portfolio applications". They cite examples including STINMOD to model the distributional impacts of taxes and benefits (Percival et al. 2007), TAXSIM to compare federal tax policy proposals on mortality (Kim 2018), and Health&WealthMOD (Schofield et al. 2009) to capture the economic impacts of health and changes in health status across multiple government portfolios and the national economy. By harnessing such hybrid and cross-portfolio MSM applications, public health researchers may capitalize on existing tools and generate more robust estimates of the impacts of the social determinants of health.

References

Ballas, D., Clarke, G., Dorling, D. et al. (2006). Using geographical information systems and spatial microsimulation for the analysis of health inequalities. *Health Informatics Journal* 12 (1): 65–79.

Basu, S., Seligman, H., and Bhattacharya, J. (2013a). Nutritional policy changes in the supplemental nutrition assistance program: a microsimulation and cost-effectiveness analysis. *Medical Decision Making* 33 (7): 937–948.

Basu, S., Glantz, S., Bitton, A., and Millett, C. (2013b). The effect of tobacco control measures during a period of rising cardiovascular disease risk in India: a mathematical model of myocardial infarction and stroke. *PLoS Medicine* 10 (7): e1001480.

Choi, S.E., Seligman, H., and Basu, S. (2017). Cost effectiveness of subsidizing fruit and vegetable purchases through the supplemental nutrition assistance program. *American Journal of Preventive Medicine* 52 (5): e147–e155.

Commission on the Social Determinants of Health (2008). *Closing the Gap in a Generation: Health Equity through Action on the Social Determinants of Health. Final Report of the Commission on Social Determinants of Health*. Geneva: World Health Organization.

Cordova, A., Girosi, F., Nowak, S. et al. (2013). The COMPARE microsimulation model and the U.S. Affordable Care Act. *International Journal of Microsimulation* 6 (3): 78–117.

Edwards, K.L. and Clarke, G.P. (2009). The design and validation of a spatial microsimulation model of obesogenic environments for children in Leeds, UK: SimObesity. *Social Science and Medicine* 69: 1127–1134.

Egger, M., Smith, G.D., and Sterne, J.A. (2001). Uses and abuses of meta-analysis. *Clinical Medicine* 1 (6): 478–484.

Glied, S. and Tilipman, N. (2010). Simulation modeling of health care policy. *Annual Review of Public Health* 31: 439–455.

Gortmaker, S.L., Wang, Y.C., Long, M.W. et al. (2015). Three interventions that reduce childhood obesity are projected to save more than they cost to implement. *Health Affairs* 34 (11): 1932–1939.

Gruber, J. and Seif, D.G. (2009). *When is Health Insurance Affordable? Evidence from Consumer Expenditures and Enrolment in Employer-Sponsored Health Insurance*. Cambridge, MA: Massachusetts Institute of Technology: Department of Economics.

Hennessy, D.A., Flanagan, W.M., Tanuseputro, P. et al. (2015). The Population Health Model (POHEM): an overview of rationale, methods and applications. *Population Health Metrics* 13 (1): 24.

Kim, D. (2016). The associations between US state and local social spending, income inequality, and individual all-cause and cause-specific mortality: The National Longitudinal Mortality Study. *Preventive Medicine* 84: 62–68.

Kim, D. (2018). Projected impacts of federal tax policy proposals on mortality burden in the United States: a microsimulation analysis. *Preventive Medicine* 111: 272–279.

Koh, K., Grady, S.C., and Vojnovic, I. (2015). Using simulated data to investigate the spatial patterns of obesity prevalence at the census tract level in metropolitan Detroit. *Applied Geography* 62: 19–28.

Kristensen, A.H., Flottemesch, T.J., Maciosek, M.V. et al. (2014). Reducing childhood obesity through US federal policy: a microsimulation analysis. *American Journal of Preventive Medicine* 47 (5): 604–612.

Kypridemos, C., Guzman-Castillo, M., Hyseni, L. et al. (2017). Estimated reductions in cardiovascular and gastric cancer disease burden through salt policies in England: an IMPACTNCD microsimulation study. *BMJ Open* 7 (1): e013791.

Laditka, J.N., Laditka, S.B., Olatosi, B., and Elder, K.T. (2007). The health trade-off of rural residence for impaired older adults: longer life, more impairment. *National Rural Health Association* 23: 123–132.

Lay-Yee, R., Milne, B., Davis, P. et al. (2015). Determinants and disparities: a simulation approach to the case of child health care. *Social Science and Medicine* 128: 202–211.

Michaud, P.C., Goldman, D., Lakdawalla, D. et al. (2011). Differences in health between Americans and Western Europeans: Effects on longevity and public finance. *Social Science and Medicine* 73 (2): 254–263.

Muennig, P.A., Mohit, B., Wu, J. et al. (2016). Cost Effectiveness of the Earned Income Tax Credit as a Health Policy Investment. *American Journal of Preventive Medicine* 51 (6): 874–881.

National Centre for Social and Economic Modeling (2012). The Cost of Inaction on the Social Determinants of Health, Report no. 2. Canberra, Australia: NATSEM.

Pearson-Stuttard, J., Kypridemos, C., Collins, B. et al. (2018). Estimating the health and economic effects of the proposed US Food and Drug Administration voluntary sodium reformulation: microsimulation cost-effectiveness analysis. *PLoS Medicine* 15 (4): e1002551.

Percival, R., Abello, A., and Vu, Q.N. (2007). Model 9: STINMOD (Static Incomes Model). In: *Modeling Our Future: Population Aging, Health and Aged Care* (eds. A. Gupta and A. Harding), 477–482. Emerald Group Publishing Limited.

Pitt, A. and Bendavid, E. (2017). Effect of meat price on race and gender disparities in obesity, mortality and quality of life in the US: a model-based analysis. *PLoS One* 12 (1): e0168710.

Procter, K.L., Clarke, G.P., Ransley, J.K., and Cade, J. (2008). Micro-level analysis of childhood obesity, diet, physical activity, residential socioeconomic and social capital variables: where are the obesogenic environments in Leeds? *Area* 40: 323–340.

Robert Wood Johnson Foundation Commission to Build a Healthier America (2009). *Beyond Health Care: New Directions to a Healthier America*. Princeton, NJ: Robert Wood Johnson Foundation.

Schofield, D., Passey, M., Earnest, A. et al. (2009). Health&WealthMOD: a microsimulation model of the economic impacts of diseases on older workers. *The International Journal of Microsimulation* 2 (2): 58–63.

Schofield, D.J., Zeppel, M.J., Tan, O. et al. (2018). A brief, global history of microsimulation models in health: past applications, lessons learned and future directions. *International Journal of Microsimulation* 11 (1): 97–142.

Tam, J., Levy, D.T., Jeon, J. et al. (2018). Projecting the effects of tobacco control policies in the USA through microsimulation: a study protocol. *BMJ Open* 8 (3): e019169.

Tanton, R., Vidyattama, Y., McNamara, J. et al. (2009). Old, single and poor: using microsimulation and microdata to analyse poverty and the impact of policy change among older Australians. *Economic Papers: A Journal of Applied Economics and Policy* 28 (2): 102–120.

Thoemmes, F. and Ong, A.D. (2016). A primer on inverse probability of treatment weighting and marginal structural models. *Emerging Adulthood* 4 (1): 40–59.

Vreman, R.A., Goodell, A.J., Rodriguez, L.A. et al. (2017). Health and economic benefits of reducing sugar intake in the USA, including effects via non-alcoholic fatty liver disease: a microsimulation model. *BMJ Open* 7 (8): e013543.

Wolf, D.A., Laditka, S.B., and Laditka, J.N. (2002). Patterns of active life among older women: differences within and between groups. *Journal of Women and Aging* 14: 9–25.

Wolfson, M. and Rowe, G. (2014). HealthPaths: using functional health trajectories to quantify the relative importance of selected health determinants. *Demographic Research* 31: 941–974.

10

Section Summary

Daniel Kim

Bouvé College of Health Sciences, Northeastern University, Boston, MA, USA
School of Public Policy and Urban Affairs, Northeastern University, Boston, MA, USA

10.1   Summary of Previous Chapters

In this section of the book (Chapters 7–9), we have introduced the concepts and methods for implementing microsimulation modeling and reviewed empirical applications of microsimulation models (MSM) within the social sciences and public health, particularly as they relate to the social determinants of health.

Chapter 7 offered an introduction to the concepts and methods of microsimulation modeling in the social sciences. Verbist and Philips discussed various types of microsimulation models, presented underlying data options, and detailed the policy scope of current models. They further outlined the fundamental steps and components for constructing microsimulation models, including inputting data, developing policy rules, and validating them. Finally, they discussed applications for policymaking including health-related microsimulation models.

Chapter 8 focused on empirical evidence in the social sciences, a field in which microsimulation has played a major role ever since its inception. Figari and Lezzi summarized key approaches and applications of MSM within the fields of economics, demography, geography, transport, and environmental sciences and identified the overlap in work between these different fields and the conceptual overlap between MSM and agent-based modeling (ABM) as modeling approaches.

In Chapter 9, I systematically reviewed the empirical evidence on the use of MSM to study the social determinants of health. I further provided examples of MSM applications to other areas of study, including intermediary determinants of health and health care policy. This review revealed some common threads in applications across microsimulation studies. It also identified several important gaps in the literature that serve as hanging fruit for future MSM research.

I conclude this section of the book with a discussion of some of the policy applications of microsimulation modeling and a description of some of the remaining empirical gaps that if addressed could help to advance the study of the social determinants of health.

10.2 Direct Public Policy Relevance of Microsimulation

Similar to ABM, microsimulation has the capacity to directly influence policies under current consideration. Chapters 7–9 reviewed a number of published policy-related applications of MSM. Some notable MSM that have had real-world policy applications include the Gruber Microsimulation Model (GMSIM), which has been used to estimate the effects of comprehensive health care reform in the entire United States under the Affordable Care Act (ACA) in 2010 (Gruber and Seif 2009), and the US Congressional Budget Office (CBO)'s health insurance simulation model (HISIM), which has been employed to estimate the budgetary and coverage effects of the insurance coverage provisions of the ACA (Banthin 2016). For example, the CBO applied this model to project that the 2017 House Republican health bill to repeal the ACA would cause 23 million people to lose coverage by 2026 and drive $834 billion in federal Medicaid cuts over the next 10 years—reversing all of the historic coverage gains achieved since the ACA was enacted in 2010 (Congressional Budget Office 2017).

A second example of MSM to simulate counterfactual scenarios based on current policy discussions is a microsimulation by Mathematica Policy Research to estimate the effects of proposed changes to supplemental nutrition assistance program (SNAP) eligibility, participation, and benefits (Cunnyngham 2018). In 2018, the US Congress worked to resolve differences between House and Senate versions of the 2018 farm bill. Policy discussions about this bill included proposed changes to the SNAP. The House version (H.R.2, The Agriculture Improvement Act of 2018) of the bill would alter SNAP policies related to resources and state eligibility. Through a microsimulation analysis, Mathematica projected that nearly 2 million (roughly one in 11) households receiving SNAP benefits would lose eligibility under certain provisions of the House Farm Bill – H.R. 2, the Agriculture Improvement Act. In addition, among these households, 34% (677 000 households) included seniors, 23% (469 000 households) included children, and 11% (214 000 households) included persons with disabilities (Cunnyngham 2018). Of the households with children losing eligibility, more than half lived in poverty. Together, these striking figures suggested harmful impacts to vulnerable populations that helped to inform policymakers in policy discussions of the House bill.

A third example is the tax microsimulation analysis by Kim (2018) described in Chapter 9, which projected the impacts on mortality of modifying federal income tax structures based on proposals by two US presidential candidates in 2016: Donald Trump and Senator Bernie Sanders. Using the TAXSIM microsimulation model, this study estimated that there would be 29 689 more deaths/year and 31 302 fewer deaths/year from all causes under the Trump and Sanders plans, respectively. Under a modified Sanders plan that included higher top tax rates, 68 919 fewer deaths/year were projected. Under a modified Sanders plan with redistribution, 333 504 fewer deaths/year were estimated. As a whole, this study provided evidence to suggest that policies that both raise federal income tax rates and redistribute tax revenue could yield marked reductions in the total number of annual deaths among Americans. During the lead-up to the tax bill that was signed into law in 2017, this study garnered significant media attention and was shared over social media by Senator Bernie Sanders.

Overall, the above three examples serve to highlight how MSM can be applied to simulate alternative policy scenarios and provide highly relevant information to policymakers regarding policies under current consideration. Through informing policymakers' decisions, MSM is a potent tool with the ability to help move the needle on enacting policies to improve population health.

10.3 Bridging Gaps to Advance Microsimulation Modeling of the Social Determinants of Health

Despite the promising strides that have been taken to apply MSM to model the social determinants of health, some important MSM modeling and evidence gaps remain. We have discussed some of these gaps in the last chapter. To advance the use of MSM to model the social determinants of health, several additional gaps exist. Below, I outline these additional gaps and suggest possible paths for bridging them.

First, greater dialogue is needed between social science researchers and public health researchers who apply MSM. Currently, the International Microsimulation Association (IMA) holds an international congress on microsimulation research biannually and invites work from all disciplines. The IMA world congress is one such forum that can facilitate dialogue between researchers. Other venues such as major social science or public health meetings (e.g. of the American Sociological Association or the American Public Health Association) could also facilitate such dialogue by holding dedicated sessions for research on microsimulation modeling and health. Likewise, leading social science journals (e.g. Social Science & Medicine, the scope of which includes a wide range of health topics) could advance such dialogue through special issues of the journal on MSM and health.

Second, we need more dialogue between public health researchers who are applying different MSM approaches such as spatial microsimulation, tax micro-simulation, and disease microsimulation. Again, such dialogue could be facilitated by national, regional, or international public health meetings (e.g. of the American Public Health Association or the European Public Health Association) and related public health journals (e.g. the American Journal of Public Health and European Journal of Public Health) by designating theme issues on MSM.

Third, despite the apparent recent exponential growth of MSM as an applied methodology, training for researchers in MSM methods is still rather limited. Even among system science methodologies, other approaches such as ABM, social network analysis, and system dynamics are better known and applied in the public health sphere and have more opportunities for training (although, as mentioned in Chapter 6, even those opportunities for ABM are relatively limited).

Fourth, common sets of guidelines for reporting and sharing of program code through open access (Richiardi and Richardson 2017), implementing MSM models and using data for published analyses, and calibrating and validating MSM models are lacking. As mentioned in Chapter 9, implementing reporting guidelines for MSM research such as adapted STROBE statements could help to standardize reporting such as information on the quality of underlying epidemiologic studies and on how potential biases were specifically addressed.

Last, it is vital for MSM models to tackle critical contemporary issues, particularly those under current policy debate that have policymakers' attention. As illustrated by several key examples in this chapter, these current issues include those related to health care (e.g. the ACA) and social policies (e.g. income tax and SNAP-related policies). Such efforts to tackle current issues can help to raise the profile of MSM research as a policy-relevant discipline and thereby bring more attention and resources including additional funding to the field.

Overall, through adopting each of the above possible paths and bridging these gaps, the promises of MSM as a modeling and simulation tool to understand and influence the social determinants of health through policies and interventions may be more fully realized.

References

Banthin, J.S. (2016). Microsimulation of demand for health insurance. https://www.cbo.gov/sites/default/files/114th-congress-2015-2016/presentation/50948-healthinsurance.pdf

Congressional Budget Office (2017). H.R. 1628: American Health Care Act. https://www.cbo.gov/system/files/115th-congress-2017-2018/costestimate/hr1628aspassed.pdf

Cunnyngham, K. (2018). *Simulating Proposed Changes to the Supplemental Nutrition Assistance Program: Countable Resources and Categorical Eligibility*. Princeton, NJ: Mathematica Policy Research.

Gruber, J. and Seif, D.G. (2009). *When is Health Insurance Affordable? Evidence From Consumer Expenditures and Enrolment in Employer-Sponsored Health Insurance*. Cambridge, MA: Massachusetts Institute of Technology: Department of Economics.

Kim, D. (2018). Projected impacts of federal tax policy proposals on mortality burden in the United States: a microsimulation analysis. *Preventive Medicine* 111: 272–279.

Richiardi, M. and Richardson, R. (2017). JAS-mine: a new platform for microsimulation and agent-based modeling. *The International Journal of Microsimulation* 10 (1): 106–134.

Part IV

Conclusions

11

Future Directions

Daniel Kim[1,2] and Ross A. Hammond[3,4,5]

[1] *Bouvé College of Health Sciences, Northeastern University, Boston, MA, USA*
[2] *School of Public Policy and Urban Affairs, Northeastern University, Boston, MA, USA*
[3] *Center on Social Dynamics & Policy, The Brookings Institution, Washington, DC, USA*
[4] *Brown School, Washington University in St. Louis, St. Louis, MO, USA*
[5] *The Santa Fe Institute, Santa Fe, NM, USA*

This concluding chapter offers some vision for how ABM and MSM research may help lay the groundwork for future research on the social determinants of health. We contrast ABM and MSM and describe an empirical example of a hybrid ABM–MSM modeling approach that combines their unique properties. In this chapter, we further discuss facilitating factors and barriers to the continued emergence of ABM and MSM as modeling and simulation tools for the social determinants of health and comment on the promising implications of implementing these modeling and simulation approaches in the future.

11.1   Avenues for Future Research

The future of ABM and MSM research holds considerable promise for advancing our understanding of the social determinants of health. As we have seen throughout the main body of this book, ABM and MSM have high potential for application to the study of the social determinants of health, leveraging their particular strengths as methods to provide new kinds of insight.

As discussed in Chapter 6, ABM can be used in a variety of ways as part of a scientific research agenda in the context of social determinants of health: (i) to uncover and understand important mechanisms that lie at the core of each social determinant; (ii) to inform policy decision-making, as it has in other areas of public health, by projecting potential impacts (intended or unintended) of a variety of interventions, as well as potential trade-offs or synergy between intervention elements; and (iii) to aid in translation, scaling, or improved efficiency in the existing interventions.

As detailed in Chapter 9, future possible directions for MSM applications to the study of the social determinants of health include expanding the scope of microsimulation to other social determinants of health such as social policies and

New Horizons in Modeling and Simulation for Social Epidemiology and Public Health,
First Edition. Daniel Kim.
© 2021 John Wiley & Sons, Inc. Published 2021 by John Wiley & Sons, Inc.

integrating aspects of spatial microsimulation, disease microsimulation, health-care policy, and/or social policy microsimulation into the same analysis. For instance, spatial microsimulation that dynamically integrates microdata on demographic, socioeconomic, and macro-level policies and characteristics would better mirror aspects of the real world. Furthermore, incorporating novel methods to strengthen causal inference would be a useful complement to make more accurate projections for the impacts of modifying the social determinants of health.

11.2 Conceptual Model and Empirical Examples of Integration of ABM and MSM

Microsimulation models aggregate micro-level population data (e.g. census data) to make future projections at the population and subpopulation levels. While MSM relies on rich detailed data including on individual characteristics (e.g. demographic and socioeconomic factors) and behaviors, it typically does not simulate interactions among individuals. By contrast, ABM simulates individual interactions and feedback that can offer important insights into emergent properties at the population level.

Given their unique properties, ABM and MSM approaches offer complementary techniques that could conceivably be usefully integrated into a hybrid modeling approach for modeling complex systems and health. For example, in the United Kingdom, Modeling and Simulation for e-Social Science (MoSeS) synthesizes the UK population using census samples and various distributed microdata and then projects individuals into the future from year 2001 to 2031. By simulating discrete demographic processes at a fine spatial scale, the hybrid modeling approach of MoSeS combines the strengths of both MSM and ABM to model complex social systems. While MoSeS' modeling approach is grounded in microsimulation, it takes advantage of the agent-based modeling flexibility of constructing heterogeneous agents to model the complexity of social interactions and behavioral processes. The ease of introducing unique rules for individual agents in ABM also helps to improve the model when there is a knowledge gap or unavailability of data.

Using MoSeS, Wu et al. (2011) previously explored hypothetical scenarios of mortality projections based on the impacts of (i) current residence location; (ii) first residence location in the system/birth places; and (iii) mortality dependent on personal migration histories. In the first scenario, all individuals are simulated in an MSM. Their survivals are determined against an age-, sex-, and location-specific mortality probability generated on the basis of local information about the current location of residence. An ABM approach is used in the second and third scenarios, where agents carry their own histories along with them and have to check on such histories to determine their mortality probabilities. In the second scenario, the

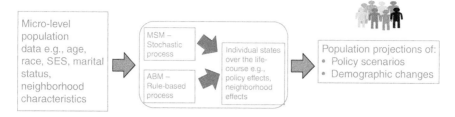

Figure 11.1 Conceptual components of a potential ABM–MSM hybrid model and its applications. *Source:* Adapted from Bae et al. (2016).

survivals are determined on the basis of the mortality rates of individual first residence location/birth places. In the third scenario, the impact of personal migration history on mortality is modeled. Mortality is projected on the basis of the mortality rates of the area where the individual stays the longest to date. Wu et al. (2011) have compared these scenarios for the population of Leeds in the United Kingdom to observed mortality and demonstrated variations in mortality projections across scenarios. Such findings show that personal history could have a significant impact on mortality. This hybrid approach could be particularly useful in future research that simulates residential histories over the life course to more validly project the impacts of social determinants on morbidity and mortality. In such a scenario, an MSM approach alone would likely be inadequate. Likewise, one could conceive of ABM rules for heterogeneous behavioral responses to social policies (e.g. welfare policy changes) that could be integrated into a hybrid ABM–MSM model. This would more accurately reflect the complex impacts of social and economic policies on households over the life course within populations.

In Figure 11.1, we show some conceptual components of a possible ABM–MSM hybrid model and the potential applications of this model to project future policy and demographic changes. Using micro-level population data, MSM (through a stochastic process) and ABM (through a rule-based process) simulate individual states over the life course and then allow us to make summary projections at an aggregate population level about the impacts of various policy scenarios and demographic changes.

11.3 Facilitators and Constraints in the Continued Emergence of Modeling and Simulation of the Social Determinants of Health

The key facilitating factors for the continued emergence of ABM and MSM include the presence of funding for research applications of systems science methods to population health. For example, in the United States, from 2011 to 2018, the National Institutes of Health allocated large research grant funding through a special emphasis grant review panel on systems science methods and health (Department of Health and Human Services 2011). The Office of Behavioral and Social Sciences Research at the NIH has also sponsored an annual training institute on systems science and health for public health research scientists, spanning agent-based modeling, system dynamics, and network science approaches.

Yet, despite the promise of systems science modeling approaches for advancing knowledge on the social determinants of health, the funding commitment at the US federal level remains rather uncertain over the long term. Furthermore, it is still uncommon for course curricula within schools of public health to include coursework on systems science methods such as ABM and MSM, unlike growing content in other methodological areas such as causal inference. This is in spite of systems thinking being one of the interdisciplinary domains relevant to contemporary public health practice that was recommended (although not required) by the US Association of Schools and Programs of Public Health (ASPPH) for Master of Public Health students in 2006 (Calhoun et al. 2008). Such funding and training commitments would likely be enhanced by additional priority setting and requirements from the top to down, for example by the US Department of Health and Human Services and the ASPPH.

The adequacy of federal funding commitments is further dependent on concomitant commitments to research on the social determinants of health. Previous research suggests underinvestments in such research. For example, although 46% or more of mortality and morbidity have been attributed to social and economic factors (Park et al. 2015), it has been estimated that only 1% of key NIH-funded research grants correspond to terms related to the social determinants of health and evidence-based methods (Kim 2019).

As discussed in Chapter 6, additional constraints for ABM to reach its full potential include issues related to data such as the current lack of guidelines for ABM modelers to help in optimizing data collection and the lack of data being more widely available that could facilitate replication. We presently lack sufficient operationalization of theories of individual behavior in ABM models as well, although emerging work on human decision-making that draws on marketing science research and noncognitive models that come from neuroscience looks promising.

As described in Chapter 10, further gaps and barriers for MSM to become more fully realized include a lack of dialogue between social science and public health researchers using MSM and between public health researchers who are applying different MSM approaches, a lack of training for researchers to use MSM, an absence of standard guidelines for reporting MSM models and data, and a need to tackle contemporary policy-related issues.

Likewise, a barrier to integrating ABM and MSM approaches includes the absence of shared dialogue between ABM and MSM researchers. This could be overcome by major public health meetings (e.g. of the American Public Health Association or the European Public Health Association) by holding dedicated sessions for research on systems science and health. Similarly, social science and public health journals such as Social Science & Medicine, the American Journal of Public Health, and the European Journal of Public Health could advance such dialogue through special issues on systems science. Training opportunities for systems science should further try to avoid siloing of single systems science approaches by jointly teaching multiple methodologies including ABM and MSM to the same audiences.

Finally, as public journals increasingly receive and review manuscripts that apply ABM and MSM approaches, the standardization of criteria for reporting (e.g. through statements for simulation studies analogous to the STROBE statement for observational studies) will become ever more important. This will ensure that journal editors and reviewers consistently and rigorously evaluate the research being performed using common standards.

11.4 Implications for Public Health

Through realizing the true potential of agent-based modeling and microsimulation modeling approaches, both individually and in combination, researchers will be much better positioned to inform public health practitioners and policymakers of the benefits and risks associated with a range of intervention and policy decisions. As a result, practitioners and policymakers will be better equipped to help achieve population health improvement and equity goals. For example, these modeling and simulation tools can enable a richer understanding of the upstream determinants of and the possible solutions for current and emerging epidemics in the United States, including the novel coronavirus (COVID-19), obesity, fatal drug overdoses, and firearm-related injuries—epidemics that threaten the average life expectancy of Americans. Through combating such epidemics with these potent modeling and simulation tools, the United States may finally reverse the tide of declining life expectancy. Indeed, while the life expectancy trend in America stands in stark contrast to trends in other western developed nations, it is far from an inevitability—and is shaped and malleable at multiple spatial levels by the ubiquitous social determinants of health.

References

Bae, J.W., Paik, E., Kim, K. et al. (2016). Combining microsimulation and agent-based model for micro-level population dynamics. *Procedia Computer Science* 80: 507–517.

Calhoun, J.G., Ramiah, K., Weist, E.M., and Shortell, S.M. (2008). Development of a core competency model for the master of public health degree. *American Journal of Public Health* 98 (9): 1598–1607.

Department of Health and Human Services (2011). Systems science and health in the behavioral and social sciences (R01). https://grants.nih.gov/grants/guide/pa-files/PAR-11-314.htm

Kim, D. (2019). Bridging the epidemiology-policy divide: A consequential and evidence-based framework to optimize population health. *Preventive Medicine* 129: 105781.

Park, H., Roubal, A.M., Jovaag, A. et al. (2015). Relative contributions of a set of health factors to selected health outcomes. *American Journal of Preventive Medicine* 49 (6): 961–969.

Wu, B.M., Birkin, M.H., and Rees, P.H. (2011). A dynamic MSM with agent elements for spatial demographic forecasting. *Social Science Computer Review* 29 (1): 145–160.

Index

New Horizons in Modeling and Simulation for Social Epidemiology and Public Health,
First Edition. Daniel Kim.
© 2021 John Wiley & Sons, Inc. Published 2021 by John Wiley & Sons, Inc.

Wiley Series in Modeling and Simulation

Mission Statement

The *Wiley Series in Modeling and Simulation* provides an interdisciplinary and global approach to the numerous real-world applications of modeling and simulation (M&S) that are vital to business professionals, researchers, policymakers, program managers, and academics alike. Written by recognized international experts in the field, the books present the best practices in the applications of M&S as well as bridge the gap between innovative and scientifically sound approaches to solving real-world problems and the underlying technical language of M&S research. The series successfully expands the way readers view and approach problem solving in addition to the design, implementation, and evaluation of interventions to change behavior. Featuring broad coverage of theory, concepts, and approaches along with clear, intuitive, and insightful illustrations of the applications, the Series contains books within five main topical areas: Public and Population Health; Training and Education; Operations Research, Logistics, Supply Chains, and Transportation; Homeland Security, Emergency Management, and Risk Analysis; and Interoperability, Composability, and Formalism.

Advisory Editors • Public and Population Health
Peter S. Hovmand, Washington University in St. Louis
Bruce Y. Lee, University of Pittsburgh

Founding Series Editors
Joshua G. Behr, Old Dominion University
Rafael Diaz, MIT Global Scale

Homeland Security, Emergency Management, and Risk Analysis

Forthcoming Titles

Zedda • Risk and Stability of Banking Systems

Interoperability, Composability, and Formalism

Operations Research, Logistics, Supply Chains, and Transportation

Public and Population Health

Arifin, Madey, and Collins • *Spatial Agent-Based Simulation Modeling in Public Health: Design, Implementation, and Applications for Malaria Epidemiology*

Kim • *New Horizons in Modeling and Simulation for Social Epidemiology and Public Health*

Forthcoming Titles

Hovmand • *Modeling Social Determinants of Health*

Training and Education

Combs, Sokolowski, and Banks • *The Digital Patient: Advancing Healthcare, Research, and Education*